KITTY CAMPION'S

HANDBOOK OF
HERBAL HEALTH

KITTY CAMPION'S

HANDBOOK OF
HERBAL HEALTH

LEOPARD

Note

This book gives non-specific, general advice and should not be relied on as a substitute for proper medical consultation. The author and publisher cannot accept responsibility for illness arising out of the failure to seek medical advice from a doctor, or a registered medical herbalist.

This edition published in 1995 by Leopard Books
Random House, 20 Vauxhall Bridge Road,
London SW1V 2SA

ISBN 0 7529 0049 8

Set in Melior

Printed and bound in Great Britain by
Mackays of Chatham PLC, Chatham, Kent

Contents

To Jill Davies and to my students for whom my respect, affection and concern are boundless.

Introduction

I'm painfully aware that half the world is starving but it is equally obvious that obesity has become an epidemic in the West. This is a different kind of malnutrition, but nevertheless it *is* malnutrition, a peculiar form of starvation induced by ingesting empty calories, that is, food with no nutritional value at all. In January 1983 the Royal College of Physicians of London confirmed that, in common with people in the USA and other Western countries, the British, particularly the young, are getting fatter but are actually eating less in terms of quantity than their ancestors fifty years ago. The burning question is not so much the quantity but the quality of the food we eat.

The average Western refined diet is so poor that it cannot hope to supply us with all we need for positive glowing health. Real food is rapidly becoming an endangered species. Almost ninety-eight per cent of everything we eat passes through the hands, or more generally the machines, of food processors. Yet in this country there is only one qualified nutritionist to approximately every seventeen food companies.

The problem is not so much what is taken out of our food but what is added. Chemical additives by way of stabilisers, colouring, extenders, preservatives and antioxidants rank high on the list. Fifteen years ago food additives covered by formal regulations numbered 2,703 and the applications for permission to use still more continue to deluge the government. Not many of these have been tested for safety simply because of the enormous numbers involved. Most of us eat three or four pounds of these additives every year. Many of us are intensely susceptible to them. The small print on the label of many convenience foods admitting to a 'permitted colouring' or 'permitted antioxidant' covers a multitude of sins. Take the latter by way of example: two of the antioxidants which are widely used to prevent fats and oils from going rancid, butylated hydroxyanisole (BHA) and butylated hydroxytoluene (BHT), are cumulative. That is, they are easily stored in body fat if eaten in substantial amounts – and they are present in virtually all manufactured foods containing any form of fat. BHA has been proved to upset the proper functioning of the intestinal muscles. BHT is believed to increase levels of fat and cholesterol in the blood, to induce birth abnormalities, stunted growth and baldness, liver and kidney damage and noticeable changes in brain chemistry. The UK Standards Committee has twice recommended that neither antioxidant be used in food, yet it is still widely used in many of the convenience foods which contain fat, except for baby food.

Many of us unwittingly eat enormous amounts of sugar, averaging fifty-two kilos each year. You might expect to find it in soft drinks, but it is also present in some brands of frozen peas and the manufactured muesli which many people eat so contentedly imagining it to be a 'health food'. And have you ever thought how much sugar there is in an average-sized bottle of coke? A tablespoon! More than enough to depress the ability your white blood cells have to engulf and destroy bacteria for hours. Certainly enough to begin the long slide downhill to tooth decay. The fact is we don't need any sugar. It contains no additional nutrients. (Even brown sugar is simply unwashed white sugar and contains only traces of some minerals which are more abundantly available from other sources.) It is full only of 'empty' calories. The ubiquitous fizzy drink also contains acidifying agents, salts and buffering agents, emulsifiers, carriers like ethyl alcohol, foaming or anti-foaming agents, synthetic vitamin C, caffeine and of course chemical preservatives. You may well consider yourself better off drinking water were we not currently embroiled in the controversy about the right of local authorities to add fluoride to our water supplies.

These depressing facts are only the tip of the iceberg. Chronic incapacitating degenerative disease is actually on the increase. Certainly we are living longer, but what's the point if the price so many of us pay is continuous pain? I believe the only way to combat these problems is to educate people about food so they can choose and enjoy diets which are non-toxic and complete. One of Hippocrates' first principles was 'Your food should be your medicine and your medicine your food', and the advantage herbs have is that, unlike chemical medicines, they can be incorporated into everyone's diet as preventative medicine.

But no amount of herbs will help you unless you first get your diet right. We can all participate in our own health care at this most basic level and indeed we must, because few GPs are interested in what you eat. Trying to sort out the pros and cons of sound nutrition is like trying to navigate your way through a minefield and you'll receive no help from those government bodies you may have thought had your interests at heart (the DHSS and the Ministry of Agriculture, Food and Fisheries) or from the colossally self-interested food manufacturing industry. A report in the *Sunday Times* (3 July 1983) investigating the four-year battle in Whitehall over Britain's calamitous dietary habits stated unequivocally 'anyone who eats the *average* British diet is in danger', and it looks as though the suppressions and evasions of complacent government ministers, a supine Department of Health and powerful lobbyists will perpetuate this situation indefinitely, aided and abetted by the advertising industry.

Have you noticed how during the 1970s emotive words like 'natural', 'rich and nourishing' and 'country goodness' came flooding into advertising copy in an attempt to exploit the nostalgia of what is fondly remembered as the good old days, when Victorian fathers presided over a table groaning with Nature's bounty? The reality of those days was quite different, as Flora Thompson recalls so evocatively in *Larkrise to Candleford*. But herbs did play a larger health-giving part in the diet then, even if only for reasons of poverty, because they were free. 'Good yarb beer' made with 'the finest yarrow that grew beside the turnpike' was drunk copiously by everyone, including children, and an abundance of watercress was eaten in the spring. Nutritional deficiencies would certainly have been much more widespread without the use of such natural physic.

There's a modern tendency for people to regard their bodies as machines and treat them with less respect than they afford their cars. At least their cars are generally serviced on a regular basis! And what of the soul, the spirit, the personality? Modern medicine tends to concentrate on anatomy and symptoms, and the non-physical side of a person, if it is taken into account at all, comes a very poor third. It seems that almost forty per cent of those who seek medical help have nothing physically wrong with them at all. Yet the average doctor's skills do not embrace those of counsellor, teacher and priest, nor can they be expected to shoulder this heavy burden. This is not a new problem. More than 2,000 years ago Socrates, on his return from Thrace, observed, 'because they do not study the whole patient the cure of many diseases remains unknown to the physicians of Hellas.'

Modern science might well try to reduce us and the universe to a level on which everything can be encompassed and explained by our five physical senses, but the more we discover in scientific terms the more we find there is to know.

Patients cannot be standardised, nor can their medicines, if they are to be truly effective. Which presents the pharmaceutical industry with an enormous problem, even supposing it were not antipathetic to herbal medicine as currently it is. The nature of the beast dictates that it produce drugs in huge quantities, but the problem is that the recipients of such drugs remain, thank goodness, stubbornly individual and this has led, over the years, to widespread disillusionment with modern drug therapy. One man's aspirin is another man's stomach ulcer.

Even doctors are becoming increasingly worried about the numbers of their patients being exposed to such irrefutably useful drugs as antibiotics, not just through prescription but because they are widely used in animal feed-stuffs and the end product is eaten by humans. In view of this constant barrage people are, not surprisingly, becoming immune to antibiotics. So much so that there are some within the medical establishment who are worrying about the day when antibiotics are remembered only as a 'temporary and historical' form of treatment. It seems we are now only some three years ahead on drug research and development in this area. Too small a lead for comfort. This overexposure to drugs has resulted in a peculiarly modern malady, iatrogenic illness, which is disease brought about by medical treatment. Apparently some ten to eighteen per cent of all hospital patients suffer from unpleasant side-effects caused by drugs. Goodness knows how many more of those that attend doctors' surgeries are in the same quandary.

There is an alternative to this – herbalism. But before it is wrongly elevated to the status of universal panacea, I should point out it is the chemical bastardisation of the properties of herbs that has, in many instances, led to iatrogenic disease in the first place. Many people fail to realise that conventional medicine is firmly rooted in herbalism. They tend to assume, if they think about it at all, that all those multicoloured pills have nothing to do with nature, whereas medical science still depends strongly on plant life to provide the blueprint for much modern medicine. Pharmacy tends to be more reliable because it enables chemicals to be reproduced in accurate doses and, given appropriate storage conditions, such medicines remain the same yesterday, today and for ever. But the advantages of science are limited. It is the pharmacologist's concern to extract the exact chemicals from a plant which will cure a specific disease, and these chemicals tend to be very potent because they are so concentrated. Once inside the body they have an ungovernable habit of travelling to various parts they are not supposed to be treating. The result can be side-effects which are alarming and may even be harmful.

It is here that the herbalist's use of the whole herb rather than simply a few of its concentrated chemical constituents comes into its own. For the use of the whole plant, balanced as it is by many other constituents, is altogether milder and more gentle, avoiding the toxic side-effects of its chemical cousins. The herb *Ephedra sinensis* (not to be muddled with the American species of ephedra called 'desert tea') is a good example. It is a natural source of the drug ephedrine used to help asthmatics, but used in this form it also raises the blood pressure. Fortunately, the plant itself, ephedra, contains norephedrine and pseud-ephedrine which have a slightly antagonistic effect to ephedrine, so buffering its action. Thus asthma can be helped using a remedy based on the whole plant without upsetting the patient's blood pressure. The Chinese have used ephedra, known by them as *Ma Huang*, for centuries for precisely this purpose. Digitalis and rauwolfia are among the growing list of herbs which are now proved to benefit from the balancing action of their many chemical constituents, enabling the body to cope better with the natural plant in its whole state.

And all this is not forgetting the point I originally raised that herbal remedies have the advantage over chemical ones in that they can be tailored to a patient's needs. Not for the first time nature can be seen to have many of the best answers.

The principle that underlies all alternative therapies is that there is an energy inside every human body which science is unable to quantify or explain. Herbalists call it the vital force which inspires the body to life and is chiefly concerned with maintaining its equilibrium. If this delicate balance, this homoeostatis, can be encouraged, the whole person will enjoy good health. If it is disturbed the result is disease. So a herbalist's well-rounded approach to medicine treats the patient, not the disease. It is the approach Plato advocated two thousand years ago.

> 'The cure of the part should not be attempted without treatment of the whole, and also no attempt should be made to cure the body without the soul, and therefore if the head and body are to be well you must begin by curing the mind: that is the first thing . . . For this is the great error of our day in the treatment of the human body, that physicians separate the soul from the body.' *Chronicles 156e*

A good herbalist is concerned not merely with the symptom of a disease but more importantly with finding out why the body has not been able to heal itself. Even orthodox medicine acknowledges that an astonishing number of ailments are self-limiting. Herbalists try to direct the vital force by encouraging it with herbal remedies which stimulate the body's own defences to produce the desired return to positive health. The remedies they use are individually tailored to the patient's needs, so that two patients with the same disease may be treated with quite different prescriptions, simply because the under-lying causes of a disease may be quite different in each individual.

What people now seem to forget in their headlong pursuit of the 'countrified' and 'natural' is that herbs are in fact powerful chemical factories. Their enormous nutritional and medical value comes from the presence of the many complex chemical substances in them which herbalists call their active principles. The advantage that herbs have over man-made chemicals is that nature sensibly packages her chemicals in such well-balanced and minute amounts that their safe assimilation by the body is assured. While chemical medicine is used solely to suppress disease, herbalists use nature's chemicals to stimulate the body's inherent healing powers. By reaching right down to the cause not the symptom they ensure a gradual return to full recovery. Chemical medicine seems much more spectacular, superficially at least, because it produces such quick results. But by merely blocking out the symptoms it fails to achieve a real cure, and if the illness is chronic and needs prolonged treatment the build-up of powerful chemicals in the system over a long period reaps some horrid dividends.

At this point you may be asking, what is a herb? I use the term to embrace any plant which is useful to man or beast. I include animals because they can teach us a lot about herbs. They have not yet lost their amazing instinct for self-medication. It has been estimated that one in seven of all plants have medicinal and curative properties. I think the number could be higher – our current research has only revealed the tip of the iceberg. So plants which are useful include mosses, liverworts, fungi, some of the plants we now call fruit or vegetables, algae, all those plants we commonly spurn as weeds which grow wild, as well as the more obvious cultivated herbaceous plants. Because my subject is health, I'm restricting myself to herbs with preventative or curative properties but of course herbs are stunningly versatile. They are breathtaking in their beauty and complexity, not least because their medicinal action is the result of the combined effect of many components. A single herb is a chemical factory containing a whole complex of these healing principles. Take sage, for example. Its leaves contain an essential oil which is both antiseptic and fungicidal, and tannin which is astringent. Sage tea is a disinfectant because of the combination of the essential oil and the tannin, and this synergistic action makes it an excellent gargle for sore throats. But once the tea is *swallowed*, depending on its temperature, other properties come to the fore, preventing heavy night-time feverish sweating and stopping lactation in nursing mothers. Sage also contains a toxic ketone as part of its essential oil complex which, if drunk regularly over a long period of time, produces an emmenagogic effect in women, that is, it causes spasming of the womb and may result in an abortion if the woman is pregnant. A brief look at the varied action of this one herb shows just how subtle herbal medicine is.

The majority of illnesses can be helped by herbalism. Illnesses fall broadly into those which are self-limiting because they tend to get better in time without any help, chronic conditions which fluctuate but never seem to clear up entirely, those caused by various types of stress, and a small twenty per cent which are the result of an actual acute medical condition. It is only the last category which may fail to benefit from herbal medicine, but even here herbalists believe they can help if they can catch such serious conditions early. Not that I'm decrying the benefits of modern medicine. I'd be the last one to refuse surgery for an ectopic pregnancy, but then all surgery is not necessarily of the life-saving variety. Much of it could be avoided by the intelligent use of preventive medicine, and it is here that herbalism could prove so useful. A good herbalist is very much concerned with prevention. The problem is that most patients, in my experience, do not consult a herbalist until the damage has been done and very often as a last resort, having dragged themselves from one specialist to another hoping for what increasingly becomes a 'miracle cure' as their condition deteriorates.

So this book begins with preventive medicine. The first chapter covers the basic prerequisite of a good diet without which positive health is impossible. Use the next two chapters, which expand on the micro nutrients that make up such a diet, as reference to augment the first chapter or to expand on the specific nutrients in a certain herb. Having completed the groundwork you will then be in a position to follow the simple step-by-step guide in Chapter 4 on how to prepare herbs for medicinal use (with a brief word on growing your own herbs) or, if you are unable to do this, where you can buy them. Chapter 5 lays out a programme for basic good health. Chapter 6 shows easy ways of using herbs to help with various types of stress. Chapter 7 deals with children's problems. Chapters 8 and 9 cover adult health problems beginning with small niggles and going onto more serious conditions. Chapter 10 deals exclusively with those health problems encountered by women, and the last chapter covers the problems we encounter as we grow older.

If all this advice comes too late because you're already seriously ill with, say, diabetes or heart disease, then you should seek the help of a qualified medical herbalist. You can find such a person by contacting the organisations listed in the appendix.

It is not necessary to have any knowledge of herbs to benefit from reading this book. Indeed it is specifically written for ordinary people, the aim being to help you to help yourself intelligently and enthusiastically.

I want to teach in a way that is entertaining, absorbing and accurate, believing, as I do, that such education can only lead to the active pursuit and promotion of good health. Don't misjudge me. I am by no means a 'back to nature' fanatic nor do I regard herbalism as a universal panacea. I would prefer to encourage a mingling of the knowledge and talents of the synthesist and the naturalist so that we could all benefit from the larger view without missing out on minute truths. I would like to see preventive health care enjoying at least an equal footing with modern interventionist medicine.

I am not overly starry-eyed about the future. It may take two or three generations before the much ridiculed alternative therapies like herbal medicine are accepted by the current medical establishment – not as poor and somewhat simple second cousins, but as complementary and respected partners. China has instigated a marriage between traditional and preventive medicines and modern medicine with considerable success, each therapy acknowledging the specific areas which the other copes with best. When I was there I saw the two approaches working well together. This success is largely the result of teaching people how they can best look after themselves. It is partly economics which has forced them into this synthesis, but in view of the current state of our Western economies we would do well to investigate their example. People need to be weaned away from their overdependence on their doctors as writers of prescriptions, and doctors in turn need to emerge from the barrier of the mystification behind which many of them take refuge. I may not see such a startling change of attitudes in my lifetime but it is a fight worth fighting. Once won it means we can all enjoy a standard of health which has hitherto been only a dream.

CHAPTER 1

'Let Food Be Your Medicine'

I'VE BEEN eating a natural diet as free as possible from chemical additives for so long that, when I raise the subject in a book like this, I often wonder whether I'm preaching to the converted. But then I stand in a supermarket queue and see other people's baskets groaning with processed food, chemical cleaners and empty calories. Yet it is possible to enjoy the convenience and cheapness of supermarkets and still shop wisely. My own basket is laden with fruit and fresh vegetables, good wine, mineral water, bottled juices, unsalted butter, and fresh fish. My pulses, grains, vegetable stock cubes, honey, spices and herbs (at least those I don't grow) I tend to buy from a wholefood shop where turnover is fast, quality high and prices cheap, though if you keep your eyes peeled it is possible to buy all of these from a well-stocked supermarket.

And why, you may ask, shouldn't you continue to indulge in your favourite fry-ups, plenty of white bread, fat, dead pig, and baked beans? Simply because you'll be starving yourself of the essential nutrients your body so badly needs to remain healthy. Denis Burkitt, famous for his championing of fibre in the diet, suggests 'the modern Western diet is a first-class menu for disease'. Dr Williams of the University of Texas has stated quite clearly that supermarket produce is likely to be deficient in vitamin B_6, magnesium, vitamin E, vitamin C, folic acid, and trace minerals. He goes on to say: 'All these and other nutrient items are needed to keep the cells and tissues of hearts and blood vessels healthy. Mental retardation, dental disease, arthritis, alcoholism, and possibly even cancer can be blamed on poor internal environments which the cells and tissues of our bodies have to live with. These ... can be vastly improved by nutritional means. Because of decades of indoctrination, many physicians will automatically pooh-pooh the idea that nutrition can be so important for the prevention of disease. This is because they are so inexpert in the area of nutritional physiology.' And sadly they are. The average medical course of five years touches on nutrition for a fortnight, if the student doctor is lucky. So really it is up to you to educate yourself about sound nutrition.

The Soil Association define wholefood as an 'unrefined food to which nothing has been added and nothing taken away'. Fruit and vegetables fall into this category, but then you're confronted by the problem of finding them unwaxed and unsprayed. Food can also only be as good as the soil on which it is grown, so that food grown on deficient soil, though it may look all right, is bound to be deficient in certain vitamin/mineral requirements. Eight fluid ounces of freshly-squeezed juice from a recently picked orange will provide 130mg of vitamin C, but when that orange is picked green, packed, shipped, marketed, and often finally stored on a warm dining-room table, its vitamin C content may be no more than one-third of what it was. In *Let's Eat Right to Keep Fit* Adelle Davis cites the example of a carrot which, when analysed, was found to contain no carotene at all! Yet it looked yellow, gleaming and inviting.

With any type of plant the greatest loss of nutrients occurs in shipping, canning, storing, freezing, and finally cooking. Hence my constant strictures in Chapters 2 and 3, especially as far as water-soluble vitamins are concerned. The general rule should be: if you can, grow your own, pick it fresh and eat it as soon as you can, raw. If you can't grow your own, try and buy from the best possible sources, get it home quickly and store it coolly.

What is a balanced diet?

We're far too protein-mad in the West and we adore our sugar, salt and fat. Besides which we eat 4 lbs of additives a year – that's the equivalent of twenty aspirin-sized tablets daily. A more balanced diet is one high in fibre, not just from bran and wholegrains, but from the highly complex cellulose substances in plants, one which is low in animal fats, salt and sugar, low in other additive substances like caffeine and tannin, and includes only very moderate alcohol.

The body should be eighty per cent alkaline and twenty per cent acid. Most people have extremely acid bodies because they eat an overabundance of acid-forming foods. Eggs, coffee, toast

and marmalade make for an all-acid breakfast; the conventional
meat, two veg, and steamed pud and custard an all-acid lunch.
Alkaline foods are **all** the fresh fruits and vegetables. I stress all
because some people think that citrus fruits are acid because
they have a saliva-stirring tang. They are not. The only alkaline
proteins are plain yoghurt, pumpkin, sunflower and sesame
seeds mixed in equal proportions (bonded together they contain
all eight amino acids, making a complete protein), and sprouted
seeds. Grains, cheese, fish, nuts, and eggs are all acid, as are
meat, certain cooked foods, coffee, tea, chocolate, chemical
drugs and stress, which releases lactic acid into the bloodstream.
There is nothing essentially wrong with acid foods. I'm not for a
moment suggesting you live off only raw vegetables and fruit
(though a few days of that would do you the world of good). The
only problem with acid foods is that most of us eat too much of
them.

Protein

Protein is of central importance in the diet, but the food industry
presents it as some sort of elixir, urging us to eat more and more.
Yet if you do this it will simply be wasted. Indeed, the minimum
protein intake now recommended by the World Health
Organisation has dropped dramatically over the last thirty years.
A full-grown adult officially requires less than 1¼ oz or 36 grams
of protein daily, which is much less than a two-year-old was said
to need in 1948.

When we eat more protein than we need (and most Westerners
eat 150 per cent more than the daily requirement), the body has
to work very hard to burn it up, putting extra strain on the liver
and kidneys. Some of it may be incompletely digested and the
poisonous by-products cause headaches, mucus and circulatory
problems. If you're a breakfast eater, try and eat a third of your
protein at breakfast to boost blood sugar levels and give you
strength for the rest of the day. If, like me, you can't bear
breakfast, sip a glass of fruit juice and take a tub of yoghurt and
some nuts into work to have during your mid-morning break.
Try not to eat later than 7 pm. All that heavy protein will cause
indigestion and insomnia.

And what of the quality of that protein? This is a complex
consideration. All proteins consist of chains of hundreds,

sometimes thousands, of amino acid units, which are the body's building blocks. A healthy body can easily convert some of these amino acids into other kinds of amino acids, so by and large it can utilise all the amino acids it ingests, provided there are enough of them. But there are eight, and in the case of children nine, essential amino acids the body cannot synthesise. We are also unable to store excesses of amino acids, so we must have all the kinds we need made available more or less at one sitting. If any of the essential amino acids are missing, the process of growth and reparation of wear and tear is held up and eventually the other amino acids are pushed out of the body and wasted. In order to ensure this does not happen we need to eat a mixed and varied diet. So combinations of oatmeal and milk, beans and tortillas, or beans on toast have a sound physiological basis.

Let me explain why. Those proteins which provide all the essential amino acids in correct proportions and adequate amounts are called complete proteins. Meat tends to contain an excess of essential amino acids, so the most efficient way to eat it to modify this excess and ensure its proper assimilation is by combining it with proteins like beans or cereals, or vegetables which are partially complete. Such proteins are placed in this category because they contain unbalanced proportions of the amino acids, which are present in amounts that will support life ` not encourage growth. Lastly there are proteins which contain amino acids which cannot support either life or growth and are called incomplete proteins.

Herbs fall into the partially complete category, but by combining them with complete sources of food it is perfectly possible to make up complete proteins. There are many advantages to this. Meat is expensive. Animals manage to convert plant protein into their own muscles – which we then kill and eat – only very slowly, retaining a mere five to ten per cent. More graphically, we in the West use half the world's supply of cereals and feed seventy per cent of it to our animals. (This for only about one-third of the world's population.) By contrast the Third World, which contains the remainder, feeds only ten per cent of its share of the world's cereals to animals. Our prodigality with meat in the West is nothing short of scandalous. We need to demote meat from its current prima donna role in our diets to one where it acts as a garnish, at the same time raising our intake of staples, among which I include herbs.

A herb like comfrey, for example, contains thirty-five per cent protein, the same percentage as soya beans and ten per cent more than hard cheese. What is more, it is rich in various trace minerals and in Vitamin B$_{12}$, which strict vegans who do not touch animal products miss out on. A deficiency of this vitamin will eventually result in pernicious anaemia. Of course comfrey, like all other herbs, has to be supplemented with amino acids from other sources to provide complete protein value, for the reasons I've explained.

Meat and dairy products

Meat putrefies in the intestines. The supportive tissue, that is, meat from the leg and muscle of any animal, is hard to digest. Meat strips calcium from the system and is rich in uremic acid, setting up conditions which may lead to arthritis, gout, rheumatism, bursitis, and heart problems. Beef, pork, battery chickens and turkeys contain antibiotics, hormones and other drugs. Even baby lambs are protected with chemicals against fluke worms. Animals killed in a slaughterhouse are full of adrenalin through fear, and their blood turns particularly acid. If all this hasn't put you off and you simply must eat meat, choose, if you can find them, free-range chicken, game birds, or liver and kidney of lamb, and if you're desperate for red meat, eat any other part of the lamb, which at least has the small saving grace of being relatively free from antibiotics.

Yoghurt is the most easily digested protein and is also, with other cultured milks, the only alkaline animal food. It encourages the production of benign intestinal flora in the lower colon. These help digestion and also manufacture B vitamins, in particular folic acid which is important for the proper assimilation of other B vitamins, such as B$_{12}$. The flora are destroyed by antibiotics and many other drugs, an over-acid diet and indigestion tablets. If you eat yoghurt, you should take at least 12 oz in one sitting because some will be killed by stomach acids. This may seem a tall order, but less won't work if it is being used to implant benign flora in the colon. Honey, any form of sugar, and all fruits except bananas, will also kill the culture.

The problem with yoghurt is that it forms a lot of mucus in the body, as do all dairy products except unsalted butter which should be used moderately. Milk and milk products are not well metabolised by the body because they neutralise hydrochloric acid, forcing the stomach to work overtime, and because the mucus they generate in the intestines, sinus and lungs builds up to form an impermeable coat which leads to poor absorption of nutrients, eventually resulting in chronic fatigue. If you don't believe me and you have a constant phlegm problem or sinus trouble, try cutting out all dairy products for a couple of months and see what happens. I often challenge my patients with this and they're amazed and delighted with the results.

An excellent way of weaning yourself off dairy products and getting them flushed out of the system is to eat four medium grapefruit, pith and all, evenly spaced from 8 am to 8 pm. Take four tablets of betaine hydrochloride with each grapefruit and drink only *purified* water, that is, bottled mineral water or water filtered through a water filtering jug. Start the day with an enema using purified water warmed to body temperature (see page 133) and the juice of a fresh lemon. If you feel terrible during the day, take another one. Retain it for twenty minutes if you can.

Allergy to milk, especially as far as children are concerned, is well established, and more seriously, by irritating tissues, milk tends to worsen a person's resistance to other allergens. Some recent work at the Hospital for Sick Children in Great Ormond Street, London, showed that sixty-seven per cent of children suffering recurrent migraine attacks were allergic to milk and, of this group, all but one also reacted to cheese. Children and adults have a great deal of difficulty digesting casein in milk, whereas human milk's primary protein is lactoalbumin, which babies generally assimilate easily. The same goes for calcium in cow's milk which does not metabolise properly, unlike the calcium in human milk. There are other excellent sources of easily assimilable calcium (see Chapter 3: calcium, page 95). It seems that twenty-five per cent of the babies fed on cow's milk before six months will develop one or more allergies, and the figure is much higher for those babies bottle-fed from birth. The best alternative if mother's milk is not possible is goat's milk, as soya milk does not have enough iron and calcium for babies' needs.

There is also an excellent alternative to yoghurt made from milk, which ensures the proper production of acidophilus in the lower colon.

This is rejuvelac which is a water ferment made from grains. The reaction between the grains, water and the surrounding air forms benign bacteria which, when drunk, ensure that the colon is well populated with acidophilus bacilli. These create an acid medium in the intestines, ensuring that unfriendly disease-producing bacteria does not thrive. Once implanted, eating green vegetables and raw sprouted seeds will ensure they grow and continue their good work. Foods which destroy acidophilus are coffee, chocolate, red meat and too much cooked food. Antihistamines, penicillin and sulpha drugs also wreak havoc on friendly bacteria.

Rejuvelac is very easy to make and is especially beneficial for any intestinal disorder. It should stand in a cool room while it is fermenting, otherwise you'll get a nasty fermenting mess which smells like vomit and tastes terrible.

Making rejuvelac

Sterilise the inside of a wide-necked jug with plenty of freshly boiling water and natural soap. Add 2¼ cups of purified water at room temperature (*not* water out of the tap – the chlorine in it will kill any benign bacteria) to 1 cup of whole wheat grain. You can get this by buying bottled non-fizzy water or by using a water filter. Get your grain from a reputable supplier with a fast turnover – last year's grain won't be much good for this operation. Cover the jug with a piece of cotton muslin and leave for thirty-six hours. Without shaking the mixture, strain off the resulting brew leaving the grain behind. Put it in a sterilised, covered container in the fridge. Sip all the liquid over the course of the three ensuing meals. You can use the same grain to make further batches of rejuvelac by simply adding the same amount of water, shaking gently, and leaving for twenty-four hours. It is possible to carry out this procedure ten times in all, including the first batch. Don't throw away the grain at the end, sprout it (see page 22). Very economical!

If you're allergic to wheat or it causes mucus problems, follow exactly the same procedure with millet, but renew the seeds after only four batches, otherwise the activity of the bacteria becomes too weak to be of any real use.

The mistake most people make with rejuvelac is fermenting it at too high a temperature. Most of us live in overheated houses. When I say room temperature, I mean the temperature the room would be on a reasonable spring day. Bad rejuvelac that's 'gone over the top' tastes and smells putrid.

Rejuvelac is easier to make with a positive-electric-field unit. These are difficult, but by no means impossible, to get in this country but are widely used in the US. The unit needs to be placed within ten feet of the jug to be really effective. It works by having a powerful inhibiting effect on harmful bacteria, but leaves the benign lactobacteria to multiply effortlessly. A negative-ion enhancer is the next best thing and certainly better than no attention to negative-ion enhancement at all.

Good rejuvelac tastes slightly earthy but quite pleasant, rather like a combination of Perrier water and the whey from yoghurt (the clear liquid you often have to pour off the top, or which appears when you cut firm-set yoghurt).

Rejuvelac should be taken for at least two weeks continually over the course of one year and may be taken for thirty days without any problems. When embarking on a natural healing programme which includes a bowel cleanse (this generally takes about nine months to a year) it should be taken for eight weeks in all, four at the beginning and four at the end. It's a superb way of implanting lactobacteria in the colon.

Eggs

Eggs are high in vitamins and minerals but unfortunately they cause a lot of particularly sticky mucus in the body and are very constipating. If you want to find out just how much glue you can get from egg white, just spread some on your kitchen floor and then try to get it off the next day. If you absolutely must eat eggs, remember the lecithin in them is destroyed when you cook with fat or oil, so boil or bake them. Cooked eggs are responsible for creating inorganic sulphur in the bowel. So if you break wind and it smells like rotten eggs, remember it is, in part, just that! Raw egg whites contain avidin which combines with the B vitamin biotin and stops it reaching the blood. Besides which the albumen protein of raw egg whites may pass into the blood undigested and cause allergies (eggs rank next to milk in the list of foods children are most allergic to). If you protest and say you don't eat steak tartar, remember that many other recipes such as ice cream also use raw eggs. Battery eggs are seventy per cent lower in vitamins B_{12} and fifty per cent lower in folic acid than free-range eggs.

Fish

Fish is an excellent protein and digests easily because it has no supportive muscle. When it passes into the small intestine vitamin D is formed which is needed for bone health, calcium and sugar metabolism. It is also rich in minerals like iodine which assists the thyroid gland. Salmon, herring and mackerel are especially rich in essential fatty acid. All fish is best eaten really fresh, but if you live inland and this is impossible, I really wouldn't bother with frozen fish. Surprisingly there are no regulations on the standard of fish products, and the type of fish you get in blocks is often treated with polyphosphate solution or sodium chloride so it takes up water and subsequently weighs more. These fish blocks can be made from fish fillets or fish 'mince' – when fish skeletons and trimmings are fed through a bone separator to remove bones. Not all the bones are taken out and blood, skin, nerve fibres and belly membrane also slip through. In the process the fish loses its texture and some of its flavour and it becomes discoloured. So the manufacturers then wash it to whiten it and by doing so flush out a large proportion of the water-soluble vitamins. Innocent fish fingers are made with minced fish, skeleton and all. Large scampi are often small ones which have been minced and remoulded under pressure to make bigger scampi shapes. Prawns are generally double glazed, meaning they are sprayed twice so they take up more water. And that nice, solid looking white fish steak is usually just fish mince with added water or several different pieces of fillet stuck together. If you're forced to buy frozen fish, buy it so that it is all in one piece, head and all, so you at least know what you're getting. Also try to investigate the source of your fish. The Irish Sea is the most radioactive in the world (the result of our pollution from Windscale), and though British Nuclear Fuels continue to insist that 'you get more radiation from travelling on a jet than eating Irish Sea fish', I prefer to buy my fish from other sources.

Cereal proteins

The food value of all cereals is about the same. The only drawback is that cereal protein tends to be low in one or other of the essential amino acids, notably lysine, but the pulses are rich in lysine, so a neat way to make up a cheap complete protein is to marry up cereals with pulses, rice or chapatis and dhal, beans on toast, porridge and soya milk, beans and tortillas.

Cereal fibre may well be the most beneficial of all dietary fibres. If the grain is served whole with the bran left on, the bran itself is rich in protein and fat, while the endosperm – the part of the grain which mainly acts as a food store – has a well balanced ratio of protein to carbohydrate. Overall, today's cereals are probably an adequate source of protein for most healthy adults. The trouble is that they leave little margin for error with their delicate amino acid balance, so one would be foolish to rely entirely on cereals as the main source of protein for growing children. Cultivated grains contain about fourteen per cent protein, as opposed to wild grains which contain less.

Cooking generally raises the protein content of pulses and grains. Soya, for example, is only complete when cooked, and even soya bean sprouts need to be cooked for ten minutes before eating to avoid ingesting a trypsin inhibitor. Light cooking of all legume sprouts actually enhances their nutritional value because heat makes amino acid methionine more available.

It is essential not to fall into the trap of smothering grains with fat, salt or sugar. It may transform them into a thing of seductive beauty (witness the chocolate éclair) but it will cripple their outstanding nutritional strengths – high in fibre, low in calories and nicely balanced in protein and energy.

Pulses

So far as nutrition goes these are probably the most desirable of all foods. The humble haricot is twenty-five per cent fibre, twenty per cent protein and abundant in calories to provide energy, though by the time they've been soaked and have puffed up the calorie value is about the same as a boiled potato so one should be hard put to get fat on pulses.

The big problem is that beans cause flatulence because they contain two different forms of starch which are difficult to digest, so instead of passing through the intestinal walls and being appropriately converted they form a feast for intestinal bacteria. These split them into carbon dioxide and hydrogen, the two main constituents of the gas given off by bad eggs.

Soaking helps, and most pulses except lentils need to be soaked overnight in plenty of water. (Remember to put soaking soya beans in the fridge to stop them fermenting.) Adding two or three tablespoons of cider vinegar during the course of the last half hour's simmer also helps, as does the addition of herbs like summer savoury, coriander, rosemary, parsley, thyme, garlic, sage, basil and cumin.

Pumpkin, sunflower and sesame seeds

Equally balanced and combined, these burst with vitamins, minerals and, in the case of pumpkin seeds, androgen hormone. They are alkaline and rich in essential fatty acids like aslinoleic and linoleic, vital to the youth and health of skin and glands. They also prevent thickening of the arteries by balancing cholesterol.

All nuts and seeds are twice as nourishing raw as roasted, because heat denatures the protein and fat. Once denatured, the fat becomes rancid much more easily and this leads to the formation of free radicals, which are believed to damage the circulatory system. The definition of a free radical is rather complex. Sufficient to say it is not some kind of hitherto unknown political activist, but the result of failure of an oxidising atom to add the requisite amount of electrons to complete the set. The result is an activated molecule which has a nasty tendency to extract another electron from any electron donor which consequently becomes altered and may become pathological. So free radicals behave in the body like a wild gang on the loose, with nothing to do, spoiling for action. They are believed to be responsible for the arterial eruptions of atherosclerosis.

So the message is, if you must eat roasted nuts or seeds roast your own, dry roasting in the oven or under the grill in small batches *as needed*. Commercial processes can disguise rancidity by washing and flavouring.

Sprouted seeds

Alfalfa contains forty per cent protein, mung thirty-seven per cent, fenugreek, lentil and aduki twenty-five per cent. But that's not the end of the story. All sprouts, because you grow them yourself, are free from all the chemicals which assault most other vegetables, they're groaning with vitamins, minerals and enzymes, all of which actually increase in content as the sprout germinates. To top all this they're ridiculously cheap and easy to grow.

Simply select your seeds, wash them in a sieve and pick out any stones or broken bits, tip them into a wide-necked glass jar and soak them overnight in purified water. (Chlorine in tap water will inhibit germination.) The next morning carefully pour off the water and cover the open mouth of the jar with a piece of cheesecloth secured by a rubber band or a piece of string. *Rinse* the beans with purified water through the cloth several times daily and drain them well. I keep mine exposed to light during the entire operation on a sunny windowsill, but some like to keep them in a warm cupboard and expose them to light only on the last day to encourage the production of chlorophyll. Rinse the sprouts and store in airtight containers in the fridge. Most beans and seeds take between three and five days to grow, but it's best to keep them a further day as the B_1 in lentils, for example, only peaks on the sixth day. B_2 only appears when two tiny green leaves show and B_{12} is superabundant in mung beans and present in most other seeds, reaching its maximum on the fourth day.

Which fats and oils?

Animal foods are rich with saturated fatty acids. Vegetable oils contain both saturated and polyunsaturated fatty acids. Saturated fats are now believed to clog up the arteries, whereas unsaturated oils, if they are cold-pressed and fresh, will not. Fats are simply oils which are solid at room temperature. When they're eaten they are broken down into glycerol and fatty acids.

The body can manufacture all of the fatty acids from natural sugar, except for three – linoleic, arachidonic, and linolenic – called the essential fatty acids. These are vital for the formation of certain body substances in the brain, lungs, thymus and iris of the eye. The average Western diet is very poor in linoleic acid in particular. All vegetable oils, particularly soya bean oil, are also rich in lecithin, which helps the action of linoleic acid. (Interestingly it has also been discovered that all soya substances have a good effect on intestinal flora.) Safflower oil contains eighty per cent of this acid, closely followed by sunflower oil at sixty-five per cent. Oils high in linoleic acid tend to lower cholesterol levels in the bloodstream, particularly when coupled with the B vitamins and vitamin E. Happily, sunflower oil is also rich in vitamin E, 1 oz of seeds containing 10mg of tocopherols. But watch your sources. The hotter the climate, the less linoleic acid in the seeds. Sunflower oil from Russia is usually three times richer in linoleic acid than that from Africa.

Olive oil is particularly rich in oleic acid which facilitates the absorption of all the fat-soluble vitamins. Best to use the virgin oil sometimes called *lucca*; from the first cold pressing of the olives, which has a delicate greenish colour and smells delicious. It's also very expensive, so spare your purse and balance your nutrition by marrying it up in equal parts with safflower oil for salad dressings and cooking. Most vegetable oils, with the exception of sesame, go rancid easily so keep them in a cool larder and add a few drops of vitamin E rich wheatgerm oil to protect them from oxidation.

When oil is hydrogenated to make margarine, free radicals (see page 21) are created and these are a major cause of premature ageing. They build calcium and excessive cholesterol deposits in the arteries. Heating cold pressed vegetable oils to high temperatures also makes free radicals. Hydrogenation is the next step on from refining, in which hydrogen gas is introduced to the oil in the presence of a metallic catalyst, generally cadmium or nickel. This bonds the hydrogen onto the oil molecules so they are saturated and transformed from a liquid into a particularly unappetising plastic solid. Partially hydrogenated vegetable oil (to prevent rancidity, spattering or foaming) is made by adding propyl gallate, methyl silicone and citric acid. Vegetable shortening, like margarine, is an artificially saturated fat made from refined oil. Margarine is a travesty of butter, vegetable shortening imitates lard, only they don't need to disguise it with nice buttercup yellow. So if you must eat fat, make it unsalted butter and be sparing with it. Don't touch margarine soft or hard. Salted butter contains sodium carbonate and calcium carbonate to neutralise the salt which is put in to stop moulds growing. Best to make your own from sweet unadulterated cream – that way at least you know what's in it.

As for the raging debate about cholesterol, it is sufficient to observe that it is increasingly recognised as *not* being one of the leading factors of heart disease. It is needed by the glands, including the sexglands, and if there isn't enough, the body will manufacture more. Prolonged stress, sugar and smoking raise cholesterol levels in the bloodstream and a fat-free diet is not the way to lower them. We need natural vegetable oils to keep the gall bladder healthy, to protect the skin and to help us metabolise the fat-soluble vitamins. Besides which they come with their own built-in safety factors – lecithin and linoleic acid. Foods which are now known actively to reduce cholesterol in the bloodstream are cooked porridge, barley, kidney beans, sweetcorn and broccoli, but avoid the latter if you have an underactive thyroid.

Carbohydrates

Wholegrains, splendid in their infinite variety – wheat, barley, millet, rye, maize, oats – are best eaten raw, by which I do not mean you need to hazard your teeth by chewing them raw. Like the seeds they are easily sprouted, which makes them easy to chew, and they are high in vitamins, minerals, enzymes, protein and carbohydrate. Colin Tudge, in his superb **Future Cook**, suggests that 'the greatest single nutritional disaster of the past 100 years in Western countries has been the decline of bread – in its nutritional quality, and in particular its fibre content; in its texture, from robust to vapid; in its flavour; and in the amount people eat.' Dr Wilfred Shute points out that the epidemic in heart disease in the West in this century can be traced back to the new steel-milling process begun in 1879, which separated the germ from the wheat kernel so that all the vitamin E and many other essential nutrients were lost. A hundred years ago the average intake of vitamin E was 150 international units (IUs). The average processed Western diet now contains only about eight IUs. If you want to put back some of the vitamin E into your diet, eat stoneground flour and make your own bread. Wholemeal or wholewheat bread may well contain all the additives permitted in white bread except bleach. If in doubt, ask. Your lovely little local baker might be just as guilty as a big supermarket chain. Pre-packed bread will have the contents written on the plastic bag. Bread 'hot from the oven' will need careful investigation.

Gluten

A lot of people restrict themselves to wheat flour which is rich with a sticky protein called gluten. This lends it an elastic resilience which makes it extremely versatile, at least as far as leavening is concerned, but gluten also sticks to the walls of the intestines, slowing down the passage of food. A lot of sticky gluten in the diet may slow down the passage of food in the intestines by a week or more and, as the food begins to putrefy, poisons absorbed from the gut into the body cause headaches, skin complaints and degenerative diseases. Gluten also tends to encase the B vitamins and stop their absorption. So if you feel you may be one of the many individuals who is highly susceptible to gluten, be imaginative with your baking and use other flours like rye and buckwheat, or mix maize, rice and potato flour together to make up a complete protein, or try soya flour. You could even try potato flour with barley which makes a delicious bread. If you're not sure how you react to gluten, try cutting it out of your diet for four weeks, then eat a thick sandwich and see how you feel. Your body will soon let you know. Rita Greer's **Gluten Free Cooking**, published by Thorsons, contains some excellent wheat-free and gluten-free recipes and the Cantassium Company make a special range of suitable flours called Trufree.

Sugar

Most people eat 5 oz of sugar daily, a phenomenal 120 lbs a year. Our endocrine systems are designed to deal with the relatively slow absorption of glucose from sugars naturally diluted in fruits or vegetables. Refined sugar gives the body a sugar rush, going straight into the bloodstream and raising the blood sugar level very fast. The pancreas re-balances the blood by removing the sugar into storage over to the liver in the form of glucose, and a much-sugared body will eventually result in a trigger-happy pancreas which pushes out insulin at the slightest pretext. The body feels sluggish and constantly in need of a boost, so that the hypoglycaemic reaches for yet more sugar and becomes trapped in a vicious circle as the blood sugar level pitches wildly up and down while the beleaguered pancreatic cells puff away in an exhausting effort to keep pace.

We all know that sugar left on the teeth causes tooth decay (in spite of a hilarious little book put out by the sugar industry extolling the virtue of sugar called *Sweet Reason*), but not many people realise that sugar also strips calcium from the body which is then deposited in joints, muscles, arteries and various other organs. Many skin infections and internal fungi such as thrush are certainly worsened by sugar eating, and all viruses, bacteria, and fungi feast in a sweet skin, as do insects, including mosquitoes. Brown sugar is fractionally higher in B vitamins and minerals than white sugar, but it is still not recommended.

Unfortunately, most of us have a natural craving for sweet things, perhaps engendered by the sweetness of breast milk or because vitamins and minerals in their natural form taste sweet, as in the form of fresh or dried fruits and young vegetables. There are suitable alternatives to sugar – maple syrup, honey, and black strap molasses, but condoning these is not a license to go mad. Use them sparingly.

Molasses

This is a by-product of the sugar-refining industry and is rich in vitamins and minerals. The darker the colour, the richer the nutritive value. Darkest of all is black strap and it is marketed under that name. It is particularly rich in inositol (lack of it causes hair loss), and next to yeast is the richest source of B_6. It is best used in cooking or added to hot drinks. Taken from the spoon it will stick to teeth and cause tooth decay.

Honey

As with molasses, the darker the better. As the bee has already pre-digested the nectar, the sugars are already converted into a form readily available to the body and easily digested. Unlike sugar, honey does not cause blood sugar to rocket to higher levels than can easily be catered for by the body. I've noticed that even babies fed on herbal teas with a touch of honey as part of their breast milk routine rarely develop colic, which is presumably because rapid assimilation stops fermentation and consequent irritation of the lining of the gut. The kidneys handle honey with much more alacrity than sugar, and honey has a very gently laxative effect as well as some value as a sedative.

Best of all, honey is a natural antiseptic and antibiotic and it is hydroscopic, meaning it draws water out of the air which makes it a good dressing for cracked, sore skin.

When using honey to cook, use only three-quarters of the amount specified in the recipe in place of sugar. If adding to liquid as part of a recipe, reduce the liquid by a fifth for each half-cup of honey used. If you keep liquid measurements the same the result will be a sloppy mess. Keep honey well covered and store at room temperature to stop it crystallising.

Maple syrup

Maple syrup is the excrescence from the maple sugar bush, and the real thing is increasingly hard to find. At the beginning of the century, nearly five million gallons a year were produced. Now the figure has dropped to one million, yet it is much more in demand and the food industry has responded by producing maple-flavoured corn syrup to fill the gap. So be a hawk-eyed label reader and make sure that what you buy is 100 per cent pure maple syrup. As it is less sweet than honey, some people prefer it in herbal teas.

Artificial sweetness?

Do not use saccharin or cyclamates. They are composed totally of artificial chemicals. If you're one of those who've indignantly protested that you don't eat 5 oz of sugar a day, look to the hidden sugar in your diet. Even some frozen peas have added sugar. Chocolate is a more obvious candidate and it is doubly damaging because it contains caffeine and a substance which causes headaches by constricting capillaries. Try carob instead, and if you really have a sweet tooth, add black strap molasses or honey. Don't leave any sugar on your teeth, not even one of the natural alternatives. Brush them after eating or, in an emergency, chew sugar-free gum.

Salt

It is essential for the maintenance of proper blood volume and pressure, for the regulation and passage of water both in and out of the body, for the transmission of nerve impulses, and the contraction of the heart and other muscles. The problem is we eat too much. We need *no* free salt in our diet at all. We get all we need in fresh vegetables, and as usual nature balances the sodium/potassium ratio beautifully in almost all of our greenery – one part of sodium to five of potassium.

Potassium/sodium balance

Sodium and potassium are finely balanced and act synergistically in the body. Everyone has precise requirements for sodium together with potassium, and the balance between the two in the body fluids maintains the osmotic pressure in a state of equilibrium inside and outside the cells.

If you take too much salt, it will overload the system with sodium and predisposes the body to high blood pressure, arthritis, and water-logged tissues such as cellulitis. Salt deposits are often found behind frequent colds, hay fever and other allergies. While giving up salt you can use a salt substitute like Ruthmol or Selora and increase the potassium-rich foods (see page 102), or better still, use natural flavouring like herbs, cayenne, garlic. Salt is also addictive. It stimulates the adrenals, forcing them to produce more adrenaline. We need only 3g a day (that's about a quarter of a teaspoon). Anyone living in intense heat or doing strenuous physical work under burning sun temporarily needs more.

Salt is ubiquitously present in most processed food and many drinks, even things you wouldn't suspect like cheese, custard powder and beer. If you eat a bowl of cornflakes followed by eggs and bacon, marmite and salted butter on toast, you'll have already consumed about 1500 mg of salt – half your daily requirement. Salt also appears in many of the 400 or so additives in our food (monosodium glutamate, etc), so it's not hard to imagine how we can manage to ingest 20 or 30g a day.

Herbs in the salt-free diet

I'm often asked which herbs to use with what foods instead of salt. For those who can't bear porridge without salt, try adding freshly minced apple mint leaves, one tablespoon to two-thirds cup of oats, and 1½ cups water. In the winter, substitute a level teaspoon of dried mint.

Vegetables are enhanced by basil, chervil, chives, borage, marjoram, oregano, parsley, summer savoury, and lemon thyme; the lighter meats, if you use them, by dill, garlic, leeks, lemon's balm, rosemary, sage, shallots and tarragon. Sweet cicely, apple and spearmint, bergamot mint, borage, and the petals from marigolds, cowslips, roses, nasturtiums, lavender flowers, and various seeds – sesame, caraway, poppy, anise and coriander – all enhance desserts.

This is not a rigid demarcation; some of the things I've recommended for savouries will go with sweet dishes and vice versa. You need to experiment and use a subtle blend of discrimination and imagination. For example, I use sweet cicely liberally with its exquisitely silky, deliberately sweet anise-flavoured leaves, spreading them as an edible platter on which I lay my strawberry or cucumber salad. Basil I use sparingly as it has a pungent, peppery flavour, and a couple of fresh leaves is usually enough, except in the case of pesto when it is used by the handful.

It matters too at what stage you decide to add herbs to your food. Heat can either increase or destroy flavour. Prolonged gentle simmering releases the aromatic substances in the herb without frittering too much away into the atmosphere. Hard, fast boiling tends to drive off the more volatile flavour of herbs, but increases the overall taste by concentration.

Fruit

All fruits are alkaline and cleanse the body beautifully, particularly if eaten with the skins intact and well washed: much of the goodness of most fruit lies in the skin or just beneath it, so don't peel it. A whole apple – skin, well-chewed pips and all – is much richer in magnesium than apple juice and, if you can bear to eat a lemon with its skin, the amount of B and C vitamins, protein, iron and potassium more than doubles. Freshly picked off a tree is the best way to eat fruit (make sure it hasn't been sprayed first); otherwise patronise a discriminating greengrocer and avoid one who puts fruit outside on the pavement where it gets saturated in carbon monoxide fumes.

Be careful with dried fruit. Apricots, pears, peaches, nectarines, and apples are generally put in sulphur houses to retain their colour and such houses fumigate the fruit with sulphur dioxide, a very poisonous gas. Raisins and sultanas are often dipped into a potassium carbonate solution before drying. The majority of commercially dried fruit is sprayed with mineral oil to make it look bright and luscious, but such oil stops the absorption of all the fat-soluble vitamins. Figs and dates are often treated with glucose which you'll recognise by its white powderiness. If the manufacturers are being honest they'll put sulphur dioxide or sulphur on the box, but if in doubt ask, and if you can't get a satisfactory answer buy where you can.

All that said, dried fruits bought from a good supplier are an excellent source of minerals and enzymes. Go for tacky, dark-looking dried fruit and ask about its origins. Fruit from Australia and California is generally dried out in the sun rather than in sulphur houses. Apricots are high in an iron which is particularly well assimilated by the body and are rich in vitamin A and copper (good when you have a chocolate craving). Dates have the highest natural sugar content of all the dried fruits, while prunes are a good natural laxative with the special ability to draw poisons through the intestinal walls from the bloodstream and flush them out through the bowel.

Vegetables

If you can, eat your vegetables raw and freshly picked while there's still life in them (see page 12). Dead food cannot create living cells. When you cook vegetables you destroy their roughage, their alkalinity and most of their vitamins and enzymes. Try a blindfold taste test on a scrubbed raw potato. It tastes a little like an apple and is an excellent blood cleanser.

Generally, the outer darker leaves and the tops of vegetables like carrot, turnip and beet, are better for you than the root and inner bleached leaves because they contain more nutrients and are easier to digest.

The worst thing you can do to a vegetable, next to boiling it to a pulp, is to freeze it, because freezing definitely destroys flavour. Try serving a bowl of fresh green peas next to a bowl of frozen ones and you'll see what I mean. Make one or two large salads a day the centre of your meals – high in fibre, low in calories, pleasing to the eye and, carefully chosen, delicious on the tongue.

Both fruit and vegetable juices, preferably fresh-pressed in a juicer or squeezed with a simple lemon squeezer if it's citrus fruit, are excellent cleansers, alkaline and bursting with easily assimilated vitamins and minerals. However, remember they do lack fibre and are a very concentrated form of nutrients so they need to be used carefully. Horseradish, watercress, garlic and other juices pressed from the more pungent herbs should be added a teaspoon at a time to other juices because they are so strong in flavour (an inbuilt warning from nature that you can have too much of a good thing). It's just possible that you can overdo parsley juice, for example, which is high in apiol, so use herbs in juices as you would do in food – gently and discriminatingly – combining the strong-tasting partner with a milder, sweeter one – parsley and carrot, tomato and watercress. Beetroot juice is a powerful liver detoxifier, cabbage juice a rich source of vitamin C and particularly good for stomach ulcers; papaya, sometimes called paw-paw, contains a protein-digesting enzyme which helps the digestion, and pineapple juice contains the meat-digesting enzyme bromelain and is particularly helpful for sore throats.

Water

Next to oxygen, water is the most important factor for survival, so use the best quality water you can get. In this country the health authorities are continuing to fluoridate water, whereas in every other European country such fluoridation is banned because it is believed to be a slow-acting poison. In 1977 the International Society for Fluoride Research at the Oxford Union produced new and unequivocal data which clearly established that artificially fluoridated water can be very harmful to some people, producing mongolism and cancer. It also inhibits the production of enzymes in the intestine, which are vital for healthy digestion.

And this is only part of the problem. Chlorine is the chemical most widely used in water to kill bacteria and the authorities are obliged to keep within certain prescribed safety limits, 0.2 to 0.3 parts per million. Sometimes they remove some of the chlorine afterwards, but when it stays behind it may trigger allergic reactions by marrying up with hydrocarbons. It also makes water taste and smell horrid. Ammonia is sometimes added to partner and so hold the chlorine in water, and sulphates (aluminium or ferric) are occasionally added to settle impurities. Consider too the way the water reaches you, sometimes by antiquated wooden systems, often by lead piping which is eaten into by acidic soft water, or more generally by copper piping which leaves heavy deposits of unwanted copper in the body.

Nitrates filter into the water wherever it is drawn from farming areas where farmers use nitrates in fertilisers. These increase the risk of methaemoglobinanaemia, a blood disease which can kill young bottle-fed babies, and nitrates *may* induce stomach cancer. Asbestos is used in some high-pressure water pipes and, if it causes cancer when we breathe it in, even in miniscule quantities, what does it do when we drink it?

Good water filters, which can be bought in the form of a jug with a carbon filter over the top or a single tap attachment, remove chlorine and heavy metal contaminants like lead zinc, and copper; artificially added fluoride can only be removed by distillation or ion exchange. If fluoride is naturally present in your water together with a balanced supply of water minerals, then I'd leave well alone. But do drink the purest water you can afford. There are two types of water filter – one you can attach to a tap, the other you pour the water through a separate filter into a jug. The Thames Valley Water Authority prefers filters which are not permanently attached to a tap because they may encourage the growth of bacteria and cause a slimy residue. You can get round this by giving a tap filter a regular heat treatment: that is, running water at 70°F or more through the filter every fortnight for five minutes. All filters need to be changed regularly depending on how often you use them. The filter in a jug servicing a family of four needs to be changed once a month, and tap filters will last from four months to a year. (The names and addresses of some good water filter suppliers are listed in the appendix, page 296). Remember that all your cells depend on having their food transported to them via the bloodstream, which needs ten pounds of water to assist circulation.

Other drinks

Coffee and tea are stimulant and acid. Coffee strips the adrenal glands of two of the B vitamins, choleine and inositol. 500-600 mg of caffeine can increase the basic metabolic rate by ten per cent. That's only six cups of a caffeine beverage daily, and if you're getting through that much you are probably clinically addicted and may be showing symptoms of coffee addiction – headaches, anxiety state, high blood pressure, hyperacidity, nausea, increased pulse rate, dizziness and insomnia. Freshly ground coffee contains 100 mg of caffeine per cup; instant coffee 80 mg, tea 60 mg, and cola drinks 40 mg per glass. The acids in decaffeinated coffee are a lot worse than the caffeine, so don't drink that either.

Dandelion coffee is a good substitute. Not the instant sort, which is sickly sweet because it contains lactose, but the dried root. You can make your own, not easily, it requires some grubbing around, but the results are worth the effort. Choose a fine November day (when the root will be at its richest with inulin) and dig up the tap roots carefully, trying not to gouge them with your spade. Shake off the surplus soil, hold under running water and scrub with a stiff brush until clean. Pat dry with a tea towel and split any particularly thick roots with a stainless steel knife. Lay them on a baking sheet and dry out in the oven at low heat. They're ready when a piece of root snaps easily. If it merely bends it still has some way to go. My Rayburn is ideal for this – I spread out the roots on the stainless steel rack above it. When I want to use the dried roots, I then roast them in a high oven till brown and mill them finely in a coffee grinder.

Dandelion coffee tastes bitter, so sweeten with honey if desired, and serve black. It is useful for cleansing and strengthening the liver, and so purifying the blood. For medicinal use, use the freshly scrubbed raw roots which are much more effective.

Jill Davies' excellent book *A Garden of Miracles* gives full guidance on tisanes. Don't forget herbs you may not have thought about like buckwheat tea made from the leaves and flowers and rich in rutin, iron, and the B vitamins; Rooibosch tea from the *Aspalanthus linearis*, rich in vitamin C and trace minerals; Bancha tea which is the twig of the tea bush and so contains no caffeine, and which is abundant in minerals. You can get Rooibosch in a health food store and many macrobiotic shops stock Bancha. Luaka and Earl Grey, if you must succumb occasionally to 'tea-tasting teas', are at least lower in tannin and caffeine.

Herbal teas for medicinal purposes must be made up in the correct proportions. You shouldn't drink water with your meals because it dilutes the ptyalin in the saliva and the hydrochloric acid in the stomach and so cripples the digestive process, but you can drink herbal teas and dandelion coffee when eating, as they actually help digestion.

Food combinations

Certain foods lumped together cause difficulties in the digestive tract. For example, the digestive processes of starch and protein are quite different and, if you eat them together, neither will be properly digested. Apart from obvious side-effects like indigestion, this may also lead to allergies. If food is only partly broken down as it passes through the body, the immune system may pounce on it as an alien and sensitise it so that, the next time that particular food is eaten, there may be an allergic reaction to it.

So learn to order your food as you eat. Eat your protein at the beginning of the meal and your starch at the end. Chew everything very thoroughly, by which I mean at least twenty times. Up to 100 times a mouthful is not too much, though the majority find it unsociable and tedious. By chewing well, any acid in food becomes alkaline as ptyalin in the saliva starts to break it down.

Protein gets trapped in the stomach for up to three hours while the pyloric sphincter (the little valve at the end of the stomach) remains firmly closed. Fruit is digested in the duodenum and needs to scoot through the stomach so it can be digested further down in the intestinal tract. So if you combine fruit and a protein, like an apple and some nuts, the fruit gets trapped in the stomach and starts to ferment. In this instance the apple will turn into a putrid version of cider vinegar, and the alcohols released may cause headaches, liver problems and gaseous indigestion. So take your fruit and fruit juices separately from the rest of your food, either half an hour before a meal or not until at least an hour after a meal. And chew everything, including juices, well before swallowing.

Having read this chapter you may be quailing at the thought of changing your diet so radically, so I'll offer you the suggestion I always offer my patients. ***Don't do it all at once*** unless you have enormously strong will-power (and if you had, presumably you wouldn't be tucking into salted snacks, chips, biscuits, alcohol, meat, dairy products, eggs, etc). Challenge yourself with one item at a time, and once you feel you have mastered the art of doing without it, set yourself another goal. I didn't, for example, give up salt, sugar, tea and coffee all at once. It took me about eight months, and I'm still cleaning up my diet. But you'll notice something very intriguing when you transfer your allegiance to an imaginative, balanced, wholefood diet. Eventually your taste buds will get sharper and fussier and you'll actually feel nauseated, and not just naughty, when you eat the things you crave. And if you don't feel sick immediately after a year or two of doing without, you'll notice you'll get a bad headache the day after a binge, or aches and pains, or a rash or bloodshot eyes, and you'll decide it's just not worth it. If I have even a taste of cheese now, I find that within an hour my sinuses are so full of mucus I can hardly breathe. And though I'm still occasionally to be found standing outside cheese shops with saucer eyes, I won't go in and buy any because I know what'll happen afterwards.

Which brings me to the subject of the smell of burning martyr flesh. Make sure, as you change your eating habits, that it doesn't pervade your house. Try not to become a fanatic. Try not to let other people's opinions bother or sway you. You eat for yourself, not for any other reason, and if you eat something you've been told is 'good', like a nice ripe mango, and find it doesn't agree with you, then leave it alone. Don't force yourself to eat things which you feel you must, otherwise you'll get tangled up with guilt and resentment and these may be harder on your body than the food. Don't go to the other extreme and con yourself into believing that what you're eating is acceptable when you know deep down it isn't. Stand up for yourself when you're eating out. Tell your hostess about your eating habits when accepting an invitation. She'll be grateful you did. There's nothing more irritating than preparing food for a dinner party only to see your guests surreptitiously rejecting part of it because they can't eat it. Most friends enjoy the challenge of a different way of cooking. Those who don't won't invite you to dinner, so you can go to a concert with them instead! If you want to eat well, you're going to have to grasp the fact that wholefood is more than a mere terminology – it's a way of thinking, a way of life, and if you act positively it's adventurous, delicious and enjoyable. When people learn, for example, that I don't eat meat, that I don't take salt, sugar or dairy products, that I won't touch eggs, they come round to my house in trepidation rather than eager anticipation for a dinner party. I'm happy to say that, by and large, they leave bubbling with relief, enthusiasm and feeling singularly well fed.

So what's the secret? Simply judicious use of ingredients, preferably fresh and in season. In winter I might start the meal with a good thick home-made soup – mushroom, pea, tomato, curried lentil – served with barley bread made from barley flour, millet and sunflower seeds and a touch of oil and wholemeal flour. If it's spring, I might begin with taramasalata, a pâté, salmon mousse, or perhaps a simple salad of sliced orange and avocado pears dressed with walnut oil and red wine vinegar, or melon, cucumber and tomatoes served with hot herb bread. If the asparagus looks good early in the summer I'll garnish it with soya mayonnaise; if the watercress is abundant I might serve iced watercress soup. Leeks with thyme in a vinaigrette dressing make an unusual starter, and if vegetables look particularly luscious I'll serve them up as crudities on a bed of ice with a creamy walnut dip kept hot on a burner. If mussels are in season I'll begin with a fragrant soup, if the field mushrooms look juicy I'll serve them hot, stuffed with plenty of mixed fresh herbs and wholewheat breadcrumbs. Or maybe I'll serve prettily shaped brown pasta shells smothered with pesto, using fresh basil, pine kernels, olive oil and *tofu* (a bean curd made from soya milk) instead of the traditional parmesan cheese. It tastes just as good! When tomatoes are really tasty, instead of being pale, watery and thick-skinned as they are most of the year, I'll serve them sliced with coriander in an avocado sauce.

The main course, even if it is entirely vegan (without animal protein or dairy products), needn't present a problem. Millet which has been casseroled and served with nuts generally goes down well. If it's hot and you want to keep things simple try *dolmades* (vine leaves, or, at a pinch, cabbage leaves stuffed with rice and herbs and simmered in tomato sauce) and served with a Greek salad. My husband makes a sensational *Biber Dolma* – a Turkish dish of peppers stuffed with onions and pine kernels. The latter may sound exotic but are readily available in wholefood shops. A rye and lentil pilau with raw tomatoes, cucumber and onion is a friendly dish on a cold winter's evening. A vegetarian chilli with lots of fresh herbs and spices has been pronounced more delicious than its meaty cousin. Curried lentils and vegetables served with brown chapatis warms even the most sceptical heart.

If it's summer and I want to serve an entirely raw menu I might begin with gazpacho, a cold tomato soup with lots of interesting garnishes, and then serve a variety of salads, perhaps Waldorf salad made with apple, celery, raisins and garnished with tahini mayonnaise made crunchy with sesame seeds. A salad using as many sprouted seeds as possible, heightening the texture with nuts and Florence fennel, is high in protein. Salads in winter need not be a problem if you use seasonal vegetables: cabbages of all hues, carrots, celery, onions, radishes, Jerusalem artichokes, turnips, parsnips, beetroot, and baby Brussels sprouts can all be dragooned into action. They are best served with a baked potato or another more exciting variation, *alu koftas*, a spicy Indian dish, or potato scones or a pear and potato casserole. Potatoes and winter salads are a complete meal in the dark days when the body craves comfortable foods.

If fish is not a problem then the varieties of fish are, of course, endless. *Teriyaki*, marinated fish which is then cooked and served with stir-fried vegetables and brown rice, has succeeded in seducing the most ardent carnivore I know. Herring in oatmeal, mackerel stuffed with gooseberries, skate in black butter, and salmon wreathed in sorrel sauce are more conventional English dishes.

Dessert is never any problem. When there's plenty of fresh fruit a home-made summer pudding oozing its purple juice through a casing of wholemeal bread tastes as spectacular as it looks. I stew the fruit in honey, not sugar. Or perhaps raspberries and strawberries piled into melon halves, or a sorbet of puréed fruit and honey served with spicy apple cinnamon biscuits. Fruit fools are easily made in advance and look pretty served with different shaped home-made biscuits. If I want to serve something really unusual I might try elderflower pancakes or gingered pears with nasturtiums, but, by and large, I think fruit is best left unsullied because that way it retains most of its nutritional content.

In the winter I might succumb to a carob orange mouse made with tahini (a sesame seed paste) and carob (a chocolate-tasting powder made from St John's locust fruit). Children and grown men who still love their nursery puddings adore chestnut cream or plum pudding made with wholewheat breadcrumbs and honey instead of suet and sugar, or fruit crumbles beefed up with coconut or oatflakes.

I tend to keep ordinary meals simple but follow the same seasonal rules. In summer breakfast might be fresh fruit, or a dried fruit compote, or Whole Earth baked beans (which are made without sugar), or freshly picked field mushrooms stewed in their own black juices with grilled tomatoes. In the winter I'll go for a home-made muesli or a raw granola, both of which keep well. Sometimes I moisten it with a nut milk made with almonds, cashews and honey puréed with water in a blender and strained. Otherwise I'll use a fruit juice. On cold mornings I'll make a good rib-sticking bowl of porridge and add sliced bananas or some muscatels, or if it's Sunday and I've got more time I might make buckwheat crêpes filled with puréed fruit, or cornmeal pancakes served with real maple syrup. Fruit or vegetable juice is my chosen drink for breakfast, though sometimes I'll have a herbal tea or a substitute coffee made from grains, figs and chicory.

Generally my lunches are raw even in winter, to ensure that at least fifty per cent of what I eat is raw. If I want bread at lunch I'll use the Essene bread I keep in the fridge made from sprouted rye or wheat grains which are then puréed and, mixed with a touch of olive oil and enough wheatgerm, are baked into a biscuit shape. The flat loaf is then baked very gently at 100°F for six to eight hours ensuring that the enzymic action is not destroyed. Slightly soft on the inside and deliciously crusty on the outside like a water biscuit.

If I have to eat out, as I frequently do at lunch time, I go for the baked or new potatoes and a salad and ask for a piece of fresh fruit. It's surprising how many restaurants will come up with this even if it's not specifically on the menu. I worry about pleasing myself first and other people second. After all, I'm the one who has to digest what I put in my mouth. Friends who know me are usually happy to cook a fish dish, and I try and appraise those who don't about my needs in advance. I restrict alcohol to meals, choosing a good white wine. Not that I dislike red wine. Unhappily it dislikes me.

I was trained as a professional cook so being creative with food comes naturally. But don't be deterred if you barely know how to scramble an egg. For one thing eggs are a thing of the past, and for another there are some excellent cookery books which will start you with the basics. Some of my favourites are:

Christopher, John Dr: *Regenerative Diet* (1983) available by mail order only from Genesis Books, 188 Old Street, London EC1, or by calling in person.

Kenton, Lesley & Susannah: *Raw Energy*. Century Publishing (1984).

Tudge, Colin: *Future Cook*. Mitchell Beazley (1980).

Petterson, Vicki: *Eat your way to Health*. Penguin, London (1983).

Walker, N.W.: *Diet and Salad Suggestions*. Norwalk Press, Arizona (1940).

Brown, Edward Espc: *Tassajara Cooking*. Shambala Berkley. London (1973).

Bateman, Michael; Conran, Caroline; Gillie, Oliver: *The Sunday Times Guide to the World's Best Food*. Hutchinson (1981).

Not all of these books steer clear of dairy products, eggs and red meat, but if you riffle through them you'll find some excellent recipes. Some, in spite of their recent publication dates, are out of print but you can still order copies through your local library, and who knows, if enough people ask it may wake the publishers up to the growing need for simple, well-constructed dietary advice.

CHAPTER 2

Vitamins

The usefulness of vitamins has recently been under attack. It has been suggested that only the very old, the poor and those on heavy drug programmes may be vitamin deficient. But I believe everyone's vitamin needs vary, and subclinical symptoms of vitamin deficiency are much commoner than we think and often very hard to detect. For example, recent research shows that twenty to twenty-five per cent of Americans and Europeans are short-of B_6 and folic acid, and the figure in Britain may be worse because we are less keen on our greens. We need to pay careful attention to the vitamin content of our diet if we are to ensure we are getting enough for positive health. The ideal balance should come through natural foods, but there are times when vitamin pills are necessary and, if this is the case, they should be natural as far as possible as opposed to synthetic. Admittedly the taking of natural vitamin pills in extremis isn't always practical. For example, a gram of vitamin C extracted entirely from rosehips means taking a pill the size of a football, because rosehip powder contains only 25-50 mg of vitamin C per 100 grams, so it would be easier to take synthetic ascorbic acid boosted with natural rosehips to ensure it works effectively.

The whole question of which foods contain which vitamins can be a minefield for the uninitiated, so the first part of this chapter explains why I feel so strongly that natural vitamins as they occur in foods are better for you than synthetic supplements, and the second part lists the herbal sources of these vitamins beginning with those which are common and easy to get hold of and finishing with those that may be new to you. Don't let the latter intimidate you. Experiment with them cautiously and you'll be surprised at how tasty and versatile they are. Some plants you can eat comfortably in large quantities like cabbage, and others, like watercress, you may only be used to using as a garnish, although there's no reason why you shouldn't try delicious chilled watercress soup and so eat much more of it. Quantity matters, of course. You'll get more vitamin C from a big heap of cabbage than you will from a garnish of watercress, but the thing that destroys the quality of food (and hence the vitamins) more than any other factor is wrong preparation and cooking methods. I caution you about these as you progress through the chapter, but I would suggest you get yourself one of the good cookery books listed on page 39 to help you further.

Natural versus synthetic vitamins

A controversy has also been raging for years about the benefits of synthetic, that is, chemically synthesised, vitamins as opposed to those present in their natural form in unprocessed food. The Food and Drug Administration of the United States insists that there is absolutely no difference between synthetic and natural vitamins – though there is one very obvious difference my palate can immediately discern and that is that natural ones taste nicer because the food they occur in generally tastes good, if well prepared.

I prefer my vitamins natural for more scientific reasons too. It is certainly true that a molecule of crystalline ascorbic acid (vitamin C) synthesised in some laboratory is chemically identical to the ascorbic acid present in a rosehip, but what the FDA seems to ignore is that the rosehip also contains vital accessory factors such as minerals, trace minerals, enzymes and coenzymes and minute traces of other important nutrients which as yet we know little about. These substances interact with each other to ensure the full absorption and utilisation of the ascorbic acid in question. They do this so effectively that practitioners who use megavitamin therapy in the treatment of their patients have found that, when they use vitamins derived from food sources, considerably lower doses can be prescribed than when using vitamins that are entirely synthetic. Herbalists have long known about this wonderful internal 'cooperation' with a single herb. The ascorbic acid present in parsley together with vitamin A, essential oils, flavones and various minerals combine to assist each other to increase the flow of saliva, cleanse the mouth and reduce the bacteria there which causes infections and tooth decay. Once in the gut, the ascorbic acid and its adjuncts are absorbed very slowly, ensuring that stools remain soft and so acting as a gentle laxative and an effective diuretic. This synergistic process may not always have been fully understood in the past, but experience has taught herbalists that verodoxin, for example, which is one of the glycosides present in foxgloves, is useless as a heart tonic if used in isolation. But add six parts of digitoxin to four of verodoxin and you have an excellent, well-balanced therapeutic tonic for the heart. Just as important is the knowledge that this combination is far safer than ten parts of digitoxin used alone, which could in fact be poisonous and have unpleasant side-effects.

Synthetic vitamins are capable of imitating some of the useful functions of the natural equivalents, but useless for others. Synthetic ascorbic acid is certainly effective as an antioxidant, but it's useless in discouraging bruising simply because it does not contain the accessory factor of bioflavenoids, present in the natural form, which actively strengthen the small blood vessels.

Natural vitamins are released in the body more gently and slowly than synthetic ones, allowing plenty of time for them to go through all the digestive processes before they are absorbed and utilised. Not only does this guarantee them through absorption but it ensures they are effectively deposited at their final destination, the body's tissues, where they appear as complex coenzymes. An interesting example of this is the difference in assimilation between synthetic and natural vitamin B_2, known as riboflavin, which is essential for cell growth and for the enzymatic reactions by which the body metabolises proteins, fats and carbohydrates. Synthetic riboflavin is digested ten times faster in the hydrochloric acid produced by the stomach than its natural counterpart. This means that most of the synthetic vitamin exceeds the kidney threshold and the overload is quickly passed out of the body in the urine. Similar quantities of natural riboflavin, in contrast, tend to be absorbed thoroughly, and very little is wasted. So too with vitamin E, where research has shown that the natural form of the vitamin is up to thirty-six per cent more active than the synthetic one, and far more potent.

Having, I hope, convinced you of the superiority of natural vitamins, let me inject a few words of caution. Don't be hoodwinked by the marketing men's jargonese. If you do need to take vitamin supplements examine the label carefully. Many vitamins labelled 'natural' contain synthetic additives combined with natural base product. So a label declaring 'Vitamin C with Rosehips' generally means the quantity of synthetic ascorbic acid dominates the presence of ground and finely powdered rosehips. If the label says 'from natural sources' this should refer to the immediate origin of the product. It should not be an attempt to disguise the many steps of organic synthesis it has taken to produce 'Vitamin A, from natural sources: dandelion leaves'. Talking of vitamin A, you may well need it to develop the hawk-like vision necessary to discriminate between 'd-alpha tocopherol', which is naturally derived vitamin E and 'dl-alpha tocopherol', which is the synthetic form of the vitamin.

Now comes the sticky question – should one be taking vitamin supplements in tablet form at all? In an ideal world, which it patently isn't, a balanced diet of unprocessed fresh foods should supply all our vitamin needs. But, as we have already seen, the real food which nourished our ancestors has undergone radical transformation by food processors who have even managed to produce completely synthetic food, so unless you are extremely conscientious about your food sources you may need to take tablets. But I should warn you when you do that most of those offered for sale as natural are, in fact, synthetic. There are many suppliers both here and in the USA who claim their products to be entirely natural when in fact they are artificial, prepared from organic compounds produced from carbon. The only vitamins available, which are naturally derived, which are at all potent are vitamin E, provided it is labelled d-alpha tocopherol acetate, and the vitamins A and D occurring naturally in fish oils.

I've found it very difficult to obtain information from manufacturers as to the base materials they use. I did discover that all commercially available vitamin C is derived from vegetable starch which is turned into glucose and then into ascorbic acid. Retinol is no longer produced using basic material from lemon-grass oil but from a very much cheaper hydrocarbon which the makers will not divulge.

So you'd better reconcile yourself to the fact that if you are taking vitamin pills whatever the label says they are almost certainly synthetic. The quality of the vitamins you eat depends on several factors.

Firstly, it matters where you live. Do you eat fresh food from your local area? Most of us don't. Is it grown organically without the aid of chemicals and pesticides? And if so, what is the soil like? Drought, continual planting, failure to rotate crops or allow for resting periods have resulted in serious soil exhaustion over the centuries, and all these factors have combined to rob us of many trace elements, particularly zinc. The first zinc-deficient people were found in Iran, Iraq and Egypt, where the soil has been cultivated relentlessly for thousands of years. The zinc levels in many parts of the Western world are now less than adequate. Signs of zinc deficiency range from anaemia, loss of taste, acne, white spots on the nail and joint pain to insomnia and emotional problems. And zinc is the only one of the sixteen trace elements we all need from plants.

Biological variability also needs to be taken into account. People living in the same area on equivalent diets have differing needs for vitamins and other nutrients. Affirming this, it was discovered after the second World War that some prisoners of war were released with only severe weight loss. Others, from the same camp and therefore presumably on the same diet, showed severe nutritional deficiencies. We still don't know enough about the upper limits of nutritional requirements, except for such obvious cases as poisoning from polar bear liver which is enormously rich in vitamin A. Yet the eskimos can, and do, eat it always mixed with other meat with impunity. We are only slowly beginning to revise our estimates of what the lower levels should be, as with protein.

The close link between optimum nutrition and health is further underlined by the fact that vitamin deficiencies inevitably occur, even among the most conscientious of us, when a person is under extreme pressure – mental or physical – during illness or convalescence, while pregnant, during the menopause.

Any form of prolonged stress may result in nutritional anaemia in susceptible people. They require increased iron, protein and vitamin B complex, particularly folic acid, vitamins B_6 and B_{12}. There is growing evidence that alcoholism may be the result of a chemical imbalance created by an inadequate diet. Though this is a chicken and egg theory because which comes first? Most alcoholics ingest empty calories in alcohol form and don't bother to eat properly. They then suffer from gross deficiency of vitamins, all of which are essential for healthy nerve functioning. This in turn may lead to a physical inability to eat properly because of a nervous reaction which impedes the swallowing mechanism. People who rely heavily on sugar-saturated soft drinks are thought to suffer from the same problem.

As the list grows, it seems almost everyone suffers from vitamin deficiencies, to a greater or lesser extent. Under no circumstances would I encourage the use of megavitamin potencies unless conducted under the watchful eye of an experienced, trained orthomolecular therapist. It is possible to poison yourself with overdoses of some vitamins, even natural ones. Orthomolecular medicine is still in its infancy, especially in this country, and sadly there are still too many self-appointed nutrition 'experts' who practise megavitamin therapy without adequate training. Megavitamin therapy is a relatively new contribution to medicine. It needs to be used carefully with consideration and respect until we are certain of its proper place in medicine. If you need the help of a properly qualified orthomolecular therapist, refer to the appendix, page 296. An experienced herbalist will certainly be familiar with the nutritional value of herbs, so for your vitamins in their natural form seek advice there too, by all means. Above all do remember when you refer to the 'How Much?' section that because all our vitamin and mineral requirements are as individual as our fingerprints my suggestions are not infallible. Adjust them for your own particular needs.

The vitamins in herbs

Vitamin A (axerophtol)

Vitamin A is not present in plants in its pure form but occurs as provitamin A (beta-carotene) which generally appears as a yellow pigment. An enzyme in our own livers is able to transform this provitamin into pure vitamin A, and it is now thought that a similar action also takes place in other organs and tissues of the body.

Carotenoids trumpet their obvious presence in many bright yellow plants, such as maize, apricots, saffron, marigolds, cowslips and golden purslane, but they also occur abundantly in green plants like parsley, spearmint and spinach.

Carotenoids may be lost by storage, leached by overcooking or destroyed by certain harmful substances present in the digestive tract. In order to avoid this it is essential that plants rich in vitamin A be picked and eaten as quickly as possible. A few hours out of the ground is half a lifetime for any delicate plant, so if you're buying them choose the freshest you can and try to stick to local plants. Lettuces flown from halfway round the world will have been out of the ground for days before they reach your table.

As soon as you get your plants home wash them briefly in cold running water. Prolonged soaking in salted water will leach out the vitamin A and many other valuable vitamins and minerals. Handle them gently. Bruising also destroys vitamins. Bear this in mind when you finally come to toss your herbs in a salad. *'Fatiguer la salade'* does not mean wear it down with sharp spoons and an aggressive arm. The process should be more like gently folding egg whites into cream.

Shake your plants as dry as you can, or pat them gently with a tea towel and place them in an airtight container or wrap them in a fresh dry cotton tea towel or brown paper. Store them away from light and air in cool conditions. Cook them as briefly as you can. The Chinese method of stir frying is ideal, or try a vegetable steamer using the smallest amount of water you can get away with without burning the pan. For details of where to buy such a steamer see page 296. Don't add salt to the cooking water. Keep the lid on tightly throughout the process and save the cooking water for soup or stock or, if there is only a trace of it, serve it up with the herbs. Blanching and freezing cause only a minute amount of vitamin loss. Canning and pressure cooking substantially drain plants of their vitamin content. My best advice is, if you can eat the plants raw, do so.

All these precautions apply to plants rich in vitamin C too, which is rapidly destroyed by exposure to heat, light and air. Copper utensils or the addition of bicarbonate of soda to the cooking water will also destroy every vestige of vitamin C.

Finally, when you come to preparing plants rich in vitamin A or C, try and break up the leaves by tearing them with your fingers. Cutting with a steel knife ensures gradual loss of both vitamins. Use wooden spoons or your fingers to toss a salad, not sharp steel spoons.

Freshness is of the essence if you are to enjoy the maximum nutritional content of any plant. Freshly picked corn on the cob needs only five to eight minutes in boiling water in order to become tender. If you leave it till the next day it will need a good half hour. If you cut the kernels off the cob they require only minimal cooking in a little boiling water and of course corn can be baked, dried and popped, or better still picked when it is young and tender and eaten raw. It tastes sweet and milky in this state, although I appreciate it may not be to everyone's taste. The tiny young kernels need a modicum of seasoning and should be chewed slowly and thoroughly, especially if you're prone to indigestion.

Sweet potatoes, both the Jersey variety and the yam, can be treated in the same way as an ordinary potato. The best way to preserve their vitamin A content (and they also contain lots of vitamin C) is to bake them in their skins. If the skins are not too tough eat these too as they're rich in mineral salts.

Yellow dock produces tender young shoots in the spring which are very palatable in a salad with a good spicy dressing to enhance their unusual flavour. Avoid the leaves later in the year. As they get older and tougher they taste terribly bitter. The young shoots can also be cooked and mixed with other wild cooked herbs like dandelion, watercress or wintercress; the resulting mixture can be perked up with some crunchy uncooked sprouts, plenty of freshly ground pepper and a knob of butter. Yellow dock is four times richer in carotene than carrots.

Goosefoot is particularly rich in vitamin A and yet we tend to feed it only to pigs and sheep, decrying it as 'pigweed' or 'dirty dick', mainly, I suspect, because it thrives on compost heaps rich in manure. The New Mexican Indians know better and prize its tender young leaves as a vegetable, and it grows widely in this country. Dandelion leaves match goosefoot as far as nutritional content is concerned, yet we persist in trying to subdue it with chemical sprays while at the same time thinking nothing of spending pounds on vitamin supplements. It's a crazy waste of money. Dandelions after all are free for the taking. The young leaves are bitter so need blanching, by which I don't mean dipping them in hot water – all you have to do is place an inverted flower pot over the plant or cover it with two slates to form a V-shaped roof. Leave the leaves protected from the light like this for ten days and then wash them, tear them up and add them to a raw spinach salad using bits of toasted wholemeal bread to complement their taste and texture. Dandelion buds are considerably less rich in vitamin A but they have a most interesting taste, rather like artichokes, and are pretty and fun to eat. Pick the white, tightly folded little buds out of the centre of the plant early in the spring. These are the parts which eventually blossom into yellow flowers. Wash them, steam them lightly and then add a little salt and a touch of yoghurt.

You can find some delicious recipes for okra in Greek or Middle Eastern cookery books and I hardly need to suggest ways in which to prepare apricots interestingly. Dried apricots are very much richer in vitamin A than fresh ones. You may not be so familiar with chard. It is a variety of spinach beet which is cultivated specially for the central rib of the leaf. Cut the whole leaf across into half inch pieces. (It's too difficult to tear.) Then steam it.

Violet leaves are astonishingly high in vitamin A. A heaped tablespoon will supply you with your minimum daily requirement. Eat the bright green leaves only, shredding them finely (scissors are easier than a knife for this). Cook them in a tiny amount of water, covering the pot tightly. You can also blanch them briefly in hot water to get rid of any slight furriness and subdue their bitterness. They taste rather like spinach but are more succulent in texture.

Nettles must be eaten young. Once they've gone to seed they taste very bitter and can be used only in a tisane. You'll have to wear gloves and long protective sleeves while you pick them, but their sting goes when they've been cooked. Like spinach they reduce down to very little so pick copious amounts.

Golden purslane marries well with sorrel in soup, and makes an interesting addition to salads if you choose only the young, succulent shoots. Marigolds and cowslips add a pretty, heart-lifting touch to any salad. Flowers have been used in salads for hundreds of years. The Elizabethans even pickled them so they would have plenty for winter. John Evelyn believed fresh flowers gave 'a more palatable relish' to salads if they were first infused in vinegar, but I find that vinegar makes them look soggy and tends to rob them of their colour which, after all, is half their delight. Use only the petals of marigolds not the centre, and

before using my own home-grown cowslips I separate them
carefully from the umbels. Don't cut them up as their tiny
tubular shape is so pretty.

What is it for?

Vitamin A is essential for the proper lubrication and maintenance of a healthy mucous membrane. This is our 'inside' skin
which stretches from the mouth right down through the
digestive system, embracing both the lungs and the sex organs.
The part which lines the lungs must have adequate moisture in
order to defend the respiratory system against invading
micro-organisms and any pollutants in the atmosphere. Vitamin
A gets used up in direct proportion to the amount of foreign
matter there is to filter out. Ozone, nitrogen dioxide and other
poisonous gases, any irritating particles and carcinogenic
material all tax the mucous membrane lining the nose, throat
and lungs, making them easier prey for infectious bacteria.
Nitrates which may be present as preservative in canned meats,
in contaminated water or in inorganic fertilisers can be
converted by bacteria in the air or in the stomach, under certain
conditions, into poisonous nitrites which inhibit thyroid
activity. We need healthy, active thyroids to convert carotene
into vitamin A.

Malfunction of the jejunum and duodenum, where most of the
conversion of carotene takes place and where it is absorbed, may
result in vitamin A deficiency. The correct utility of this vitamin
also depends on adequate amounts of fat and protein in the diet,
so slimmers must include a reasonable amount of protein in
their diets (see protein p 13) as well as some fat. Three level
teaspoons of one of the polyunsaturated oils used in salad
dressings is ideal. Constipation too often goes hand in hand with
a slimming diet, though it shouldn't if the diet is full of roughage.
You should **never** cope with this problem by using mineral oil as
a laxative, as it leaches all the fat-soluble vitamins, including
vitamin A, out of the system, and interferes with their
absorption. Children and adults absorb vitamin A more
efficiently than tiny babies and people over seventy. Diseases
like hepatitis, diabetes, colitis and cystic fibrosis also interfere
with the adequate utility of vitamin A.

Vitamin A, together with vitamin E, is necessary as a
prophylactic against ulcers. It has long been observed that

people who suffer severe injuries sometimes develop ulcers almost overnight, because all vitamin A reserves are quickly moved to the site of the injury leaving none to protect the stomach lining. Enlightened hospitals now give high doses of vitamin A on admission to prevent this.

Vitamin A is also essential for a healthy skin and is needed for the growth and maintenance of glands, bones, teeth, nails and hair. External skin conditions, particularly psoriasis and to some extent acne, can be helped by this vitamin, and it accelerates the healing of burns and wounds. Of course such conditions require a whole spectrum of vitamins and minerals as well as a cleansing diet. It won't cure anything effectively used in isolation.

The most common sign of vitamin A deficiency is night blindness. If depletion persists this may develop into softening of the cornea, ulceration of eye tissue and finally blindness.

Ninety per cent of all vitamin A is stored in the liver which is our most important cleansing organ. It works hard to filter out any harmful elements from the system before any damage can be done and leans heavily on vitamin A in its unceasing battle against toxicity. If you want to get maximum benefit from your vitamin A don't engage in strenuous activity within four hours of eating a meal rich in it.

Sources of vitamin A

The vitamin content of any plant varies according to the season. Yoghurt made from milk in summer, for example, contains twice as much vitamin A as that produced in winter because of the seasonally varying content of this vitamin in the grass. (In fact grass itself contains twenty-eight times more of all the vitamins except for D than any vegetable, and people have been known to exist on it perfectly adequately for quite long periods of time. The most famous case was that of the villagers of Auronzo in Northern Italy. In 1918 the Austrian army plundered all their food and they were forced to exist for nearly a year on grass alone. During that time everyone remained very fit and after the war they were able to return to normal food and the death rate shot up. Interestingly, during the period of this enforced mono-diet there was no ulceration of the cornea detected at all.)

In order to get some idea of how rich a plant is in carotene look at its colour. Herbs which are deep yellow or orange in colour or those with dark green leaves generally contain an abundance.

The outer green leaves contain more vitamin A than the blanched hearts. Unhappily it is generally the soft centres which taste best!

Common sources of vitamin A
The list begins with the foods richest in vitamin A:

Apricot (dried and cooked)	Broccoli
Spearmint	Carrots
Spinach	Lettuce
Watercress	Chicory
Apricots (fresh)	Corn on the cob

Less common sources of vitamin A

Dandelion leaves	Purslane
Goosefoot	Nettles
Yellow dock	Chard
Kale	Wintercress leaves
Violet leaves	Elderberries
Dandelion buds	Papaya

How much?
The official daily requirement is set at 5000 IUs with less for children and more for pregnant women and growing teenagers. Those most prone to vitamin A deficiency are children, the elderly and vegetarians. Indeed, a deficiency in this vitamin is one of the two most common nutritional deficiency diseases in the world today. In 1968 the Citizen Board of Inquiry into Hunger and Malnutrition in the United States reported that forty per cent of all Americans are deficient in vitamin A.

Nutritionists challenge the official minimum requirement, believing that it should be two to four times larger, depending on the person and the stress they're experiencing. A therapeutic dose is about 50,000 IUs daily and it is possible to take an even higher dose over a short period of time, but I must emphasise that any therapeutic vitamin treatment should be carried out under the supervision of an orthomolecular therapist: ***do not make your own decision in this area***, not least because no vitamin works in isolation to help any condition. I believe the toxic levels of vitamin A are much higher than is generally recognised. You would have to take 500,000 IUs in one dose to induce acute toxicity and doses of 20,000 IUs should be harmless even when taken over indefinite periods. But this does not give you licence to rush out and stuff yourself with vitamin A. Overdose symptoms, when the poor, overburdened liver cannot store any more, include hair loss, dry cracking skin, severe headaches and general lassitude and weakness. These don't usually manifest themselves until some six to fifteen months after the beginning of a massive intake. Toxicity is reversed within three to seven days simply by stopping the treatment. Vitamin K is also useful in the treatment of excess vitamin A, and vitamin E gives added protection against toxicity because it 'spares' vitamin A and works in close partnership with it. By final way of reassurance, there is no one food which contains enough vitamin A to cause toxicity except for polar bear liver and I've never seen that in any butcher's shop!

Vitamin B complex

The B family of vitamins is not called 'complex' without reason. For one thing it's large. What was originally thought to be one vitamin now turns out to be many. So far we've discovered thirteen vitamins in this group and there are almost certainly more waiting to be isolated. For another, like all cooperative families, each B vitamin depends on the others if it is to work properly. So you should never take the individual B vitamins in isolation (even supposing that it were possible to do so, as many tend to occur in a single food). Always rely on the whole B complex group, and then you may boost certain ones within the complex if necessary. Yeast and bran are the most reliable sources for the full B complex as it occurs naturally, but avoid those yeasts grown on petroleum products or wood pulp and choose those cultivated on hops or molasses. To ensure you are doing this if you're taking brewer's yeast in its powdered or tablet form, write and ask the manufacturer how it was made. If they ignore your question, as I've found many manufacturers do, persist until you've found a firm which is helpful.

Vitamin B$_1$ (thiamine)

The body will not store thiamine as it does A or D. Like vitamin C it is partly destroyed in the body and passes out when you urinate, so supplies have to be constantly replenished.

What is it for?

Thiamine is a vital factor in the burning of carbohydrates, fats and proteins to make energy for body processes. It has also been called the 'nerve vitamin' and is essential not only for the healthy functioning of the whole nervous system but is believed to discourage paralysis. (B_2, B_6 and E also play an important part here.) Thiamine also plays a vital role in maintaining the health of the heart and regulating its rhythm.

How much?

The official daily requirement is 10 mg, although a therapeutic dose can go as high as 100-500 mg. Children need less according to age ranging from 1-3 mg. There is no danger of overdosage as the body is very good at expelling any excess.

Deficiency of thiamine is very difficult to detect in its early stages as the symptoms are so generalised and tend to point to all sorts of other possibilities. Such symptoms may include general weakness and lassitude, weight loss and a dwindling appetite, vaguely uncomfortable feet and legs. If the situation is allowed to go on it might develop into diarrhoea alternating with constipation and possibly colitis (an inflammation of the large bowel), severe headaches and a tendency to dropsy, rough, unhealthy skin, a subnormal temperature, palpitations, wide-spread neuromuscular pathology in the form of ankle, foot, toe or finger drop and paralysis of the vocal chords. The final results will be full-blown beriberi. Of course beriberi is extremely rare in the affluent West. It is a disease which affects the poor, rice-eating population of the Third World. But thiamine deficiency to a greater or lesser degree is quite common although, as I've said, notoriously difficult to detect. People most likely to suffer from a thiamine deficiency are alcoholics or anyone suffering from diseases which impair its proper absorption, including hyper-thyroidism, severe liver disease and persistent diarrhoea. Breastfeeding mothers have an increased need for thiamine.

This vitamin is particularly susceptible to loss through heat and, as it is water-soluble, pans must always be tightly covered to prevent its evaporation during cooking. Not many of us in the West eat raw fish, but those who love *Serviche* (a Peruvian uncooked fish dish) as I do, should know that it contains thiaminase, an enzyme that destroys thiamine.

Swinging to the other extreme, a prolonged overdose can lead to B_6 deficiency as well as loss of the other B vitamins and can affect thyroid and insulin production. Indeed, it's as well to remember that prolonged ingestion of *any* B vitamin can result in significant depletion of all the others in the group.

Sources of B_1

B_1 is found in brewer's yeast and all brans (the thin external skin round all grains including buckwheat, corn, millet, oats, rice and wheat). Other plant sources are sunflower seeds, dandelion leaves, kale, watercress, broccoli, cauliflower, sweet potatoes, turnip greens, mustard cress, white goosefoot, parsnips, spinach, peas, beans and lettuce. In fact, almost all plants contain traces of vitamin B_1, but its richest sources, apart from yeast and bran, are sunflower seeds and wheatgerm.

Common sources of B_1, B_2, B_3

The list begins with the richest sources of these vitamins (with the exceptions of food listed under B_2 and B_3 separately):

Yeast	Corn on the cob
Rice bran	Cauliflower
Wheatgerm	Broccoli
Millet	Rice, brown cooked
Oats	Spinach
Sesame seeds	Sweet potato
Sunflower seeds	Lentils
Wheat	Watercress
Peas	Wheatbran

Less common sources of B_1, B_2, B_3

Buckwheat	Kale
Rye	

Vitamin B_2 (riboflavin)

Riboflavin is lost by the body through perspiration and urination. Oxygen does not harm it, nor does heat, although it is leached away in the water used for cooking because it is

water-soluble, like the rest of the B complex group. It's worst
enemy is light: milk left in the bottle and exposed to sunlight for
only two hours loses fifty to seventy per cent of its B_2 content; a
further five to fifteen per cent is destroyed during pasteurisation.
It's better to buy raw goat's milk if you drink milk at all, in waxed
cartons.

What is it for?

Riboflavin, in combination with protein and phosphoric acid,
forms enzymes which neutralise the acidity produced when
nutrients are burned up to make energy. It is essential for growth
and to maintain healthy eyes, skin, nails and hair.

Deficiencies start showing up in tiny ways at first – small
pucker lines round the mouth; a blotchy tongue, scaly, oily skin
eruptions especially in those areas where the mucous membrane
and outer skin meet, like the sides of the mouth, the nostrils and
corners of the eyes; changes in vision which produce a sort of
twilight blindness. This is somewhat similar to the night
blindness caused by vitamin A deficiency, but occurs, as the
name suggests, during the twilight hours. If the depletion
persists there may be a very painful throat with consequent
difficulty swallowing, an inflamed, cracked, burning tongue,
difficulty in walking and burning feet, and many eye problems
culminating in growth of cataracts. Very recent research
suggests that some birth defects which show themselves as
malformation akin to those produced by thalidomide may be
due to extreme deficiency in the mother, but this is far from
proven.

People most liable to deficiencies are those who are 'faddy'
about their food and won't eat certain things like green plants or
liver, those on a deliberately restricted diet as a result of
digestive disease, and alcoholics. The elderly often have greater
difficulty absorbing the vitamin because of the lack of
phosphorus in their diet or because of an inability to produce
sufficient hydrochloric acid in the stomach. Penicillin destroys
niacin, so if you're taking it increase your dosage of B_2 to 250 mg
daily.

How much?

The minimum daily requirement should be 5 mg for adults and
1-4 mg for children. Teenagers need the adult dose. A

therapeutic dose can go up to 250 mg. Fairly large amounts of the vitamin can be stored in the liver and kidneys and traces are present in the tissues.

Sources of vitamin B_2 occur generally in the same plants as B_1, and indeed most plants contain some traces of it. The only exception is buckwheat.

Vitamin B_3 (niacin)

Niacin, like riboflavin, resists onslaughts from oxygen and heat but is easily leached away in water. It occurs in almost all the body's tissues, forming oxidising enzymes which transfer hydrogen in the body's energy cycles, and its main storage centre is the liver. Alcoholics have great difficulty retaining it because of the congested state of their livers.

What is it for?

Mild deficiencies tend to show first in the tongue. It is bright red at the tip, grey and furry at the back and the breath, not surprisingly, is very anti-social. Small ulcers form on the inside of the cheeks and under the tongue. This may be followed by the dwindling of the secretion of hydrochloric acid in the stomach, and the ensuing digestive disturbance will range from indigestion to flatulence, constipation and diarrhoea. If the whole intestinal tract consequently becomes inflamed it may result in colitis.

The final outcome of a long-lasting deficiency may be pellagra and it is a horrible disease to observe, characterised as it is by what are abbreviated to the three Ds – dermatitis, diarrhoea and dementia. Fortunately pellagra is no longer as widespread as it once was, except among the very poor who are forced to exist on a very limited diet with little protein. Happily doctors have long got over their stubborn belief that this disease has long since disappeared from Western Europe and are more able to recognise it in very poor areas.

If this weren't bad enough, severe deficiencies will lead to deep depression characterised by 'crying jags'. Indeed, research which still remains highly controversial suggests that niacin can be successfully used to treat a large range of mental disorders, particularly those suffered by children, including perceptual disturbance, minimal brain disorder, hyperkiniesis, schizophrenia and autism. Given such wide-ranging claims, you can understand why many doctors remain dubious. Personally I find such research fascinating, although I'm perfectly willing to acknowledge that much more remains to be uncovered.

If you take extra niacin for therapeutic purposes you'll notice your skin flushes. Some people liken the feeling to light sunburn. Sometimes this flush leaves after a while. In other cases it recurs. The flush may be useful as far as arteriosclerosis (hardening of the arteries) is concerned, because it dilates the blood vessels, though they don't dilate all at the same time of course. This stimulating effect is subtle, ensuring there is no overall upset of the balance of the blood flow. If patients are upset by this and I am treating them for conditions other than arteriosclerosis, I use niacinamide instead. This is the non-flushing form of the vitamin.

How much?

The minimum daily requirement is 10 mg, but most nutritionists recommend up to 30 mg daily for adults and 4-15 daily for children, depending on their age.

Sources

Apart from the plants listed in the chart on page 55 (with the exception of fresh raw peas which contain no B_3 at all), niacin also occurs in reasonable quantities in sunflower seeds, parsley, dandelions, white goosefoot, mustard and cress and fenugreek seeds.

Vitamin B_5 (pantothenic acid)

The name for this vitamin comes from the Greek *pantothen* meaning 'derived from everywhere' and its naming indicates its presence in all living cells. The same is also true of B_1, B_2, B_3 and B_{12}, all of which can be found distributed throughout our bodies, but it seems that pantothenic acid is universal in its impact. It is one of the younger and lesser known vitamins and deserves a great deal more detailed research.

What is it for?

Officially so little is known about B_5 that the United States Food and Drug Administration has insisted that labels on bottles containing B_5 state 'need in human nutrition not established'. Yet much has been undertaken in the field of animal experimentation which clearly establishes the continual necessity for this vitamin.

An experiment to establish whether a deficiency in pantothenic acid altered a person's resistance to disease resulted in the volunteers complaining of weakness, burning cramps, fatigue and insomnia. The last effect was so severe that it was believed to be the cause of personality changes. Prisoners volunteering in another experiment in which they were deprived of pantothenic acid suffered from acute depression. Clearly this vitamin is one more of the links in the nutritional chain needed to prevent mental disease.

As far as resistance to disease is concerned, it was clearly established that B_5 and B_6 are essential for the production and transportation of antibodies in the blood. Without these two vitamins the chain of protection against diseases like tetanus and typhoid collapsed.

One of the most interesting things to be established about pantothenic acid is that arthritis sufferers appear to be noticeably deficient in this vitamin. It seems that some of us have an inherited need for far larger amounts of this vitamin than others. There is absolutely no indication that arthritics eat diets deficient in B_5, but rather they are deficient in **the way their bodies use this vitamin**. Researchers have found that adding cystine to pantothenic acid and administering it orally to arthritics over an eight-week period has resulted in a radical alleviation of the disease. Mind you, the treatment has to be then continued indefinitely otherwise the symptoms return. It seems that cystine is just one of the complexity of substances which helps the body to use B_5 efficiently.

Interestingly, vegetarians who eat milk and eggs (that is, not vegans) nearly always have higher levels of pantothenic acid in their blood than people who consume meat, even on a well-balanced diet.

How much?

Since our individual needs vary so greatly, this is a difficult question, but as an excess is easily flushed out of the body it is better to err on the high side, particularly if you are under stress. If rheumatism or arthritis is a problem you are advised to consult an orthomolecular therapist for advice about nutrition, as a deficiency of B_5 is almost certainly only part of the problem.

The minimum daily recommended dose has not been established (or indeed as far as the FDA is concerned even acknowledged) but I would recommend about 20-100 mg daily and a therapeutic dose can go as high as 1,000 mg.

Dry heat destroys B_5 very quickly, so bear this in mind when toasting wholemeal bread or baking oats. In canned and cooked food losses may range from fifteen to thirty per cent.

Common sources of B_5

This list begins with the richest source:

Brewer's yeast	Lentils
Peanuts	Wheatgerm
Sesame seeds	Cashew nuts
Mushrooms	Rice, brown
Broccoli	Cauliflower
Oats	Walnuts
Sunflower seeds	Wheatbran

Unusual sources of B_5

Soybeans	Kale

Vitamin B_6 (pyridoxine)

Pyridoxine ranks with pantothenic acid as one of the most recently analysed vitamins, but happily we do have a lot more information about it than about pantothenic acid.

What is it for?

The absorption, conversion and building of protein all depend on the presence of B_6. The more protein you eat the more pyridoxine you require, but as the body's metabolic demand for B_6 is increased, so the need for niacin (B_3) grows greater. I cannot emphasise enough that the body and mind are all of a piece, which means that any nutritional deficiency cannot be successfully treated simply by a single vitamin. Vitamins are all links in one long chain. If one of these links is weakened as the result of a deficiency in any single vitamin then the whole structure is in jeopardy. For complete mental and physical health we need to make sure our nutrition is perfectly balanced. In order to achieve this perfection we certainly need to take our individual capacities into account, but we should always strive towards a balance, not an overemphasis. So, in the instance of B_6, reducing your protein is *not* the way to avoid a deficiency in this vitamin. You will recall from the section about protein that your body must have it, because it then breaks down into amino acids which in turn form enzymes which are essential for the maintenance of life. Fasting with water only rapidly results in a dearth of B_6, so if you are water-fasting for more than a few days you must replace it in tablet form. We are unable to manufacture pyridoxine in our bodies so we need constantly to maintain levels orally which are right for us.

Vitamin B_6 is also essential for the correct utilisation of fats and carbohydrates, for the forming of blood and the manufacture of antibodies and hormones such as adrenalin and insulin, for the health of the skin and the hair. Its absence shows itself in a wide variety of ways from tooth decay to liver damage to the excessive production of oxalic acid which leads to kidney trouble and gall-stones and cancer of the bladder.

One of the most widely publicised findings about B_6 is that women who take oral contraceptives excrete an excessive amount of xanturenic acid and that it is possible to reverse this biochemical change by using vitamin B_6. Why worry about xanturenic acid? It is a generally useless side-product which is flushed out of the body in the urine and is manufactured from tryptophan, an amino acid which is essential for growth. If the metabolism is normal tryptophan is converted into niacin, but without B_6 the process stops abruptly, causing a B_3 deficiency which in turn just may result in schizophrenia. B_6 has also been found useful for ridding women of morning sickness and helping to alleviate premenstrual tension. Its lack can cause travel sickness, lessen resistance to middle ear infection, skin diseases, anxiety, insomnia, abdominal pain, water retention, irritability, weakness and difficulty in walking. A large number of these symptoms are part of the horrid catalogue about which women who suffer from PMT complain. Pyridoxine is also essential for warding off brain imbalances and some forms of anaemia.

This vitamin is rapidly destroyed by light and oxidation, so herbs rich in B_6 must never be cut up until a few moments before they are due to be eaten.

The people most liable to be deficient in B_6 are children and teenagers living on junk food diets who need more of it for healthy growth and development, women on the pill or those on high protein diets, those suffering from the added strains of alcohol, smoking, drugs, emotional stress and pollution. And that list more or less embraces all of us.

How much?

The minimum recommended daily allowance is 2 mg for those on a high protein diet, 1.05 mg for babies and toddlers, 2 mg for children and adults, and 4 mg for pregnant women and those who are breastfeeding. However, I believe we could all quite happily benefit from 10-75 mg daily, and a therapeutic dose could go as high as 300 mg, and 500 mg the week before a period is due.

Common sources of B_6

This list begins with the richest source:

Brewer's yeast
Black strap molasses,
   malt extract
Wheatgerm
Wheatbran
Sunflower seeds
Soybeans
Rice, brown

Tomatoes
Corn on the cob
Barley
Peas, dried
Sweet potatoes
Bananas
Peanuts
Cabbage

Vitamin B_{12} (cyanocobalamin)

What is it for?

This vitamin is perhaps best known for its highly successful use in the treatment of anaemia, but it is also vital for the healthy functioning of the nervous system, and is involved in the metabolism of fats, proteins and carbohydrates. It has the most complex chemical formula of any single vitamin, containing a metal called cobalt and phosphorous, and because of its complexity it cannot be synthetically produced. Its source is micro-organisms which exist in soil, in water, and in the digestive organs, and it depends for much of its correct functioning on folic acid.

Until the discovery of B_{12}, pernicious anaemia was tantamount to a death sentence. In its simplest terms anaemia means that a person is short of blood, not in quantity but in the essential red blood cells which carry oxygen. These cells are manufactured in the bone marrow and in a healthy person these are 5,000,000 to every cubic millimetre of blood. When the blood count falls below 400,000 red cells per cubic millimetre, the patient is diagnosed as being anaemic and will certainly feel the classic symptoms of extreme fatigue and irritability.

Red blood cells are lost by excessive bleeding. Children and teenagers also need larger amounts of these oxygen-carrying cells for proper muscle development while they continue to grow. This is why teenage girls are more likely to fall foul of anaemia than any other segment of the population.

Such simple anaemia, if neglected, leads on to pernicious anaemia, in which the nerve sheaths will be damaged and the patient may become psychotic. Unlike simple anaemia, this condition cannot be cured by adding iron to the diet because the victims lack an essential enzyme produced in the stomach and without it they are unable to absorb B_{12}. The hydrochloric acid normally produced in the stomach also dwindles, further impeding the digestive process. It is only possible to treat pernicious anaemia by injections which bypass the stomach. Patients suffering from pernicious anaemia are injected with 100 micrograms daily, for B_{12} is not toxic or dangerous even in enormous quantities.

B_{12} has been used to improve a variety of conditions, ranging from asthma, where thirty micrograms are administered daily for some months, to a displaced spinal disc, acute skin diseases and shingles, as well as, to a lesser extent, muscular dystrophy, rheumatic and arthritic diseases and osteoporosis (porous bones).

Interestingly, vitamin B_{12} is vital for the prevention of eye damage. If you simply cannot give up smoking bear this in mind. All that tobacco smoke you puff out rises upwards and injures the myelin which surrounds the optic nerve. B_{12} has been shown to help resist this. So people who have to live with heavy smokers may be cheered by this, as their need for the protection of B_{12} will be almost as great.

How much?

B_{12} is measured in micrograms (abbreviated to mcg). A microgram is 1000th of a milligram. The minimum daily recommended dose is 2 mcg for babies, up to 5 mcg for children, 50 mcg for adults, and 500 mcg for pregnant and lactating women. Vegans need 50 mcg weekly, according to Adelle Davis. Personally, I feel all of us could do well to follow her recommendation. A therapeutic dose can easily go as high as 500 mcg.

Vitamin B_{12} is sensitive to light, acids, and like the rest of its family is water-soluble, so is best eaten raw, at least as far as vegetables, nuts and fruits are concerned.

If you do feel tired, headachy, nervy and generally run down for weeks on end don't automatically assume you have a case of simple anaemia and start treating yourself with added iron and B_{12}. Consult your doctor or your medical herbalist and get a thorough examination. You may well be suffering from a simple iron deficiency, but there are other much more complex forms of anaemia, like sickle cell anaemia, which are far more serious. Not to mention pernicious anaemia, which can progress silently for years before the patient takes notice and feels creeping damage to the brain and nervous system. Take note of a statement in the *Lancet*, 9 October 1965: 'It is now generally recognised that vitamin B_{12} deficiency may be present with a wide variety of psychiatric manifestations and without anaemia or gross neurological signs: *and that these may precede the physical disturbances by months or years*' (my emphasis).

Common sources of B_{12}

There is a popular myth that B_{12} is only available in animal and dairy products and that consequently vegans need to be particularly careful about a deficiency. Actually eighty-five per cent of B_{12} in meat is lost when it's cooked, and not many people have a penchant for steak tartare. B_{12} is adequately manufactured by the bacteria in the intestines as long as they are not coated with mucus (which reduces permeability to all vitamins), and providing putrefactive bacteria – from overeating, too much protein, sugar, pollution or enzyme deficiency – isn't strongly present.

B_{12} is particularly abundant in four-day-old bean sprouts (especially mung) and can also be found in the following:

Almonds	Cabbage
Alfalfa	Corn
Apples	Comfrey
Asparagus	Dates
Bananas	Grapes
Brewer's yeast	Grapefruit
Cantaloupe melon	Pineapple
Carrots	Rice polishings
Celery	Soybean meal
Lemons	Spinach
Mushrooms	Tomatoes
Nuts	Watercress
Oranges	Water melon
Onions	Wheatgerm
Parsley	Wholewheat bread
Peaches	Peas

It is almost certainly present in many other plants which have yet to be investigated, including sea plants and algae.

Less common sources of B_{12}

These include dulse, kale, kelp, lima beans, okra and sauerkraut. B_{12} works particularly well with its companion vitamin, folic acid, found in vegetables, grains and fruits. Vegans and vegetarians can rest easy in the knowledge that it is readily available to them and should bear in mind that a properly working thyroid gland helps the absorption of this vitamin. People with healthy intestines have storage levels sufficient to maintain B_{12} levels for up to five years. Megadoses of vitamin C leach B_{12} and folic acid so if, for some medical reason you're increasing one, increase the others proportionately.

Folic acid

I list folic acid immediately after B_{12} because of the partnership between the two vitamins. Their relationship to each other is so complex that nutritionists are still not certain just how it works.

What is it for?

Where B_{12} can be used to prevent pernicious anaemia, folic acid is essential to stave off megoblastic anaemia, which is a form of anaemia in which the blood cells become abnormally large. The people most susceptible to this disease are women in the last three months of pregnancy. Many doctors now believe this particular problem is so widespread during pregnancy that they cite folic acid as the foremost vitamin deficiency. Some investigations in the United States have revealed that a folate deficiency among this particular group has been found to cover between twenty and thirty per cent of pregnant women, and if it is not immediately corrected it can produce damage to the foetus. The rate of deficiency in women with twin or multiple pregnancies has been found to rocket to an astonishing eighty per cent. In the UK B_{12} is often prescribed automatically to pregnant women.

It has been discovered also that the proper absorption of folic acid may be blocked by some types of oral contraceptives and, while this is relatively rare (the more usual causes being malnutrition, alcoholism and pregnancy), any women on the pill would do well to watch for any unusual physical or emotional symptoms. After all, the impact of oral contraception on the body's biochemical mechanisms is still a long way from being fully understood.

Folic acid is essential for the full absorption of all the other B vitamins in the intestine and seems to be concerned with bringing the blood into contact with all the body's tissues. Any digestive disorders such as sprue, coeliac disease, vomiting or diarrhoea which impair the ability to absorb food will result in folic acid deficiency. Classic symptoms of such a deficiency begin with a decrease of the normal number of white corpuscles in the blood and may include insomnia, irritability, lapses of memory, rapid weight loss, lack of hydrochloric acid in the stomach, glossitis (inflammation of the tongue) and megoblastic changes in the bone marrow.

How much?

The minimum daily recommended dose is 0.4 mg, rising to 0.8

mg for pregnant and breastfeeding women, and 0.1 mg for their babies. I feel this is rather on the low side and suggest 20 mg for adults and 100 mg during pregnancy; a therapeutic dose, supervised by a nutritionist, can go as high as 1,000 mg.

People most prone to deficiencies are pregnant women and others on badly planned diets high in carbohydrate, especially those sensitive to gluten, those living alone who tend to snack rather than plan their meals, alcoholics and people on long courses of antibiotics which hamper the absorption of folic acid.

Common sources of folic acid

These are given in descending order of quantity:

Potatoes	Watercress
Asparagus	Cabbage
Spinach	Wholewheat flour
Lentils	Peas
Turnip greens	Broccoli
Oats	Mushrooms
Avocados	Cauliflower
Lettuce	Rice, brown
Wheat	Brussels sprouts
Barley	Courgettes

Less common sources of folic acid

Lima beans	Kale
Endive	

Folic acid is easily destroyed by high temperatures. For example, spinach loses fifty per cent of its folate into the water in which it is cooked, and liver up to ninety per cent when fried. So fry your liver lightly and eat your spinach raw in salads. Folic acid evaporates readily from picked green plants kept at room temperature, so if you can't eat them immediately keep them wrapped up in the fridge. If you suspect you may be having difficulty absorbing folic acid (and it is now believed we can store it for only up to one month inside our bodies), take your folic acid in juice form. Orange juice has five to fifty times more folic acid than tomato, prune and apple juice, and three times more than grapefruit juice. Moreover, vitamin C is necessary to keep folic acid from disintegrating through oxidation. Fortunately, where it is present in green plants it is almost always coupled with vitamin C.

Biotin

What is it for?

We are not yet familiar with all the functions of biotin but we do know it is necessary for the metabolism of protein and is also involved in the biosynthesis of unsaturated fats, both processes being essential to health.

Any deficiency becomes almost immediately noticeable, showing itself in poor appetite, muscular pain, scaly dermatitis or eczema, extreme fatigue and depression, insomnia, hair loss and a susceptibility to heart and lung infections. Some nutritionists believe biotin activates lysozyme, the bacteria-digesting anti-enzyme in all the body's fluids like tears, and in mucus.

How much?

One form of biotin known as d-biotin is synthesised in appreciable amounts within the body, so there is some debate as to how much the minimum daily requirement should be. It is generally regarded as lying somewhere between 150-300 mcg and a therapeutic dose can go as high as 500 mcg as biotin is not toxic. Traces of it are present in most plants but the following are particularly rich in it.

Common sources of biotin

Brewer's yeast
Cauliflower
Mushrooms
Hazelnuts
Sweetcorn
Wholewheat
Strawberries
Bananas

It is also particularly rich in liver, so try and eat two servings a week if you can. If you're a vegetarian concentrate on yeast supplements and molasses.

Choline

We know far too little about this B vitamin, particularly in view of its vital importance.

What is it for?

So far scientists have proved that choline affects our nervous system, blood pressure, kidneys, fat metabolism and liver. So you can see why, in view of this formidable list, I stress its importance.

It is not clearly understood just how choline helps control blood pressure, and indeed exploration in this field has only been slight, but an experiment conducted in the 1950s on 158 hypertensive patients using choline relieved headaches, dizziness, palpitations and constipation within ten days. By the third week every patient's blood pressure was reduced without exception. As soon as choline was discontinued all symptoms returned. Since then it has been established that it is helpful for any circulatory disorders which are the result of hardening of the arteries. The implications of this finding are quite wide.

It means that choline is essential for the proper use of cholesterol in the body. Lecithin is a substance which the body manufactures in adequate amounts when there is enough choline and inositol (another B vitamin) present. It emulsifies cholesterol so it cannot settle on artery walls or collect as gall-bladder stones. Its importance as one of the weapons against heart disease and hardening of the arteries is therefore obvious. The richest plant source of lecithin is soybean.

The correct metabolisation of fat is also essential if the liver is to function properly. If the liver becomes clogged with fat it is unable to carry out its vital cleansing role, so eventually the whole body becomes diseased by accumulated toxins.

Choline is also important for the healthy functioning of the kidneys and as a preventative measure against nephritis. The myelin sheath which surrounds every nerve fibre is also dependent on choline. Lack of it results in an inability to control defecation and urination. Babies do not have this myelin coating and need choline to develop it before they can be toilet trained.

How much?

We are able to manufacture our own choline in the digestive tract, but in order to do so we need methionine (a protein), one of the unsaturated fats, folic acid, B_6, B_{12} and probably most of the rest of the B family. This raises an interesting point about slimming diets. If you are existing on a diet with no fat and very little protein it means the less methionine you have the harder it is for your body to manufacture choline. If you cannot manufacture choline it means you cannot make lecithin, which is one of the factors that helps to convert fat into energy. So by cutting out fat altogether and cutting right down on protein you are making weight loss much harder and slower.

According to Drs Bicknell and Prescott very little choline is excreted by the body, but they set the daily requirement at quite a high level, 650 mg. Those who take doses higher than this over a *long* period of time are liable to become deficient in B_6.

Sources

So far no government body has established a need in human nutrition for choline which seems to me somewhat ridiculous, because I believe we have managed to pervert and process our food so thoroughly that we have destroyed many of the elements necessary for the manufacture of choline. It is certainly possible to produce adequate amounts of choline on a diet rich in poultry, fresh fish, eggs, whole grains, leafy plants and seeds (particularly sunflower, pumpkin and sesame), but the average diet falls far short of this ideal balance. Besides which, we in the affluent West seem to be permanently dieting, generally unwisely.

Inositol

Even less is known about inositol than its partner choline. Certainly a combination of the two together with other nutrients is necessary for the manufacture of lecithin.

What is it for?

There is scattered and tentative evidence which suggests that inositol is useful for reducing blood cholesterol, and coupled with vitamin E it has been shown to be effective for certain kinds of nerve damage, mainly muscular dystrophy. It has been used to treat cases of baldness but is only effective in those people suffering from inositol deficiency.

How much?

Like choline no minimum daily requirement has been established, but I would recommend 1,000 mg. Inositol is destroyed by caffeine, and remember caffeine is also present in some soft drinks and in tea, not just in coffee. It is concentrated in our muscles, brain, red blood cells, in the lenses round the eye and our hearts and kidneys, which suggests that it is one of the factors necessary for a healthy heart, clear vision and mental stability.

Sources
Inositol is present in nearly all green plants in small quantities and is richly abundant in animal hearts, offal, seeds and whole grains.

Para-amino-benzoic acid (PABA)

This is a unique complex because it is classified as a 'vitamin within a vitamin' in as much as it forms an integral part of one of the B complex family – folic acid. When the sulphonamide drug was discovered in the 1940s as the first antibiotic, it was found that its chemical formula was very much like that of PABA. Consequently, when it was administered orally, the PABA in the human intestine counteracted it, and it became ineffective. As a result the FDA restricted PABA to tiny amounts in food supplements but there seems little point in such caution now that the sulphonamide drugs are so seldom used, besides which there are excellent herbal methods of combatting bacterial infection.

What is it for?
PABA is believed to be essential for the synthesis of folic acid in the intestinal tract and some scientists think that lack of folic acid leads to white hair. This is questionable as the process of greying hair is much more complex than this, enmeshed as it is in the necessity for many of the other members of the B complex family as well as copper and probably other minerals too. However, Adelle Davis, a nutritionist I greatly respect, tells us in *Let's Get Well* that she saw many instances of restoration of colour in grey hair in patients encouraged to eat yoghurt, liver, yeast and wheatgerm. Persons who take 5 mg of folic acid and 300 mg of PABA and pantothenic acid daily with some B vitamins from natural sources can usually prevent hair from greying and often restore its colour! The whole of the B complex group are necessary for healthy hair, as is the protein and lactose

in yoghurt and the vitamin E, iron, calcium and protein in wheatgerm.

Lack of PABA results in fatigue, anaemia, skin rash and hair problems. Too much can have a debilitating effect on the liver, kidneys and heart of some people.

How much?

For reasons I've already discussed, no minimum daily requirement has been established, but I would recommend 10 mg for children to be increased as they grow into adults to 100 mg daily. A therapeutic dose can go as high as 500 mg but this should not be pursued for prolonged periods of time. An orthomolecular specialist will only permit you to take such a dose under supervision for a month or two at a time.

Sources

The best sources of PABA are foods in which all the B vitamins are most abundant. Plant sources include all those listed under the B_1, B_2 and B_3 grouping.

Vitamin C (ascorbic acid)

Vitamin C is widely present in the plant kingdom, and occurs to some extent in nearly every plant. True cod roe, herring, various offals, milk and yoghurt contain traces of vitamin C, but it is predominantly a plant vitamin.

A cure for scurvy, which is the final debilitating result of vitamin C deficiency, was known but not properly understood by our ancestors. Herbalists treated the disease with remedies which included oranges, lemons and oil of vitriol (the latter, being sulphuric acid, is definitely not recommended!), scurvy grass, brook lime, cresses, parsley, chervil, lettuce, purslane, winter rocket and strawberries. *The Diary of John Manningham* (1602-3) records the following remedy: 'Of the juyce of Scourvy grasse one pint; of the juyce of water-cresses as much; of the juyce of succory, half a pint; of the juyce of fumitory, half a pint; proportion to one gallon ale; they must all be tunned together.' A very sensible solution, because scurvy grass is antiscorbutic and watercress has the added bonus of being rich in vitamin E, which cooperates with vitamin C in a mutually self-protecting role.

Some explorers (and there are astonishingly recent examples) were totally unable to grasp the principle of the necessity of fresh fruits and vegetables. Jacques Cartier, visiting Newfoundland for the second time in 1535, landed with 100 of his 103 crew almost prostrate with scurvy. A native among his men introduced him to a decoction of the leaves and bark of sassafras which wrought a cure which seemed nothing short of miraculous. James Lind later wrote: 'It wrought so well that if all the physicians of Montpelier and Louvaine had been there with all the drugs of Alexandria, they would not have done so much in one yere, as that tree did in six days.'

It was a lesson that sadly still had not been learned hundreds of years later by Scott on his voyage to the South Pole. He and his men were eventually to die of scurvy. Even the Eskimos at the opposite end of the pole knew better, incorporating into their diet, as they still do, the hardy plants and lichens which survive even in extremely cold climates. Many of these abound in vitamin C.

Vitamin C is certainly the most sensitive of all the vitamins to oxygen, light, heat, alkalis and metals such as copper. Storage is a particularly difficult problem because wherever vitamin C appears in nature it is accompanied by ascorbic acid oxidase, an enzyme which accelerates the destruction of the vitamin. As a general rule this is kept apart from the destructive enzyme in the fresh plant, but once it is picked the internal breakdown of the cells releases the enzyme and this process may be further accelerated by bruising or overhandling the plant in question. All in all, the longer the plant is out of the ground, the more its vitamin C content is dissipated. Kale loses one-third of this vitamin within the first days of harvesting and parsley about twenty per cent, so the lesson to be learned here is, if you can, grow your own.

Air destroys vitamin C rapidly. Once you've opened your canned orange juice bear in mind that 3.3 mg of ascorbic acid is destroyed by 1 ml of air, and of course shaking the juice aerates it still further. Freezing destroys vitamin C only fractionally and certainly not to any extent that should worry you. On the other hand, copper cooking implements and baking powder are lethal as far as vitamin C is concerned. Perhaps the worst culprit in this area is heat, so if you have to cook your plants keep it brief and use a high temperature to accelerate this brevity, and steam if at all possible. If you do use water keep it to a minimum and save it for adding to soups, sauces or gravies, because the vitamin C will have been leached into the water. Above all never soak, and slice and peel only at the last minute. If you have to blanch plants for the freezer, cool them as quickly as possible using cold air in preference to cold running water which will only further leach the vitamin C.

What is it for?

Vitamin C is vital for healthy bone growth, for knitting fractures and healing wounds, and for strengthening the capillaries. (People who bruise easily or suffer from nose bleeds are very likely to be suffering from fragile capillaries.) It seems that vitamin C is particularly abundant in the adrenals, the pituitary and thyroid glands, and it is essential for the efficient working of the whole endocrine system of glands and the proper production of hormones. It is also highly concentrated in the eyes and some medical reports suggest that large doses of it in the treatment of corneal ulcers have resulted in dramatic improvements. It also has a beneficial effect in cardiovascular disease, as it acts as an efficient diuretic and it helps the body to assimilate iron properly, but only if 50 mg per meal is ingested. If the dosage is any lower it has no effect at all upon the absorption of non-haem-iron.

This makes nonsense of the minimum daily recommended dose in this country of only 30 mg a day. Spread that out and it is just about 10 mg with each meal. Dosage is still a very controversial issue among nations. The Russians give their athletes 400 mg daily, the Americans recommended 60 mg and some authorities go as high as one milligram per pound of bodyweight.

How much?

Amidst all this disagreement the most important factor to bear in mind is that vitamin C is highly unstable, it cannot be stored in the body and it drains away rapidly under conditions of cold, heat, fatigue and stress. Stress is the root cause of so much disease that I have devoted a separate chapter to it (see Chapter 6). The role of vitamin C in stress conditions has been proved by the experiences of the first astronauts who were found to have very low levels of the vitamin in their bodies on their return to earth, in spite of a carefully programmed diet. It seems no one had allowed for the fact that these men, by the very nature of their jobs, were subjected to enormously high levels of stress during their flights. When this was realised the vitamin C in their diets while in space was appropriately boosted and since then there has been no further indication of lowered body levels of vitamin C.

You may be puzzled by the phrase 'body level'. This simply means the amount of vitamin C eaten determines the total quantity present in the body, which is in turn known as the body level or pool. Experiments conducted in America in 1971 determined that an intake of 75 mg of ascorbic acid daily resulted in 1,500 mg as the average body content, much of which is stored in the muscles and the endocrine system. When vitamin C was cut out of the diet altogether the body pool was drastically reduced to 300 mg after fifty-five days.

On the British daily recommended minimum dose of 30 mg daily the body pool would only be 1,000 mg, and even the most conservative researchers in this field believe that 1,500 mg is the bare minimum, while some feel 4,000 mg is a more desirable level, at which point the body tissues are saturated in vitamin C. Whether the body *should* be saturated with ascorbic acid or not is the main controversial issue between international official authorities. In fairness there is no hard evidence either way, but I do feel the British recommendation is unacceptably low because it takes no account of the widely individual variation in requirements.

I've already mentioned some of the factors that leach vitamin C from the body but consider, before you decide on your own level, two of the most commonly used drugs available today – aspirin and the contraceptive pill. How often do you take aspirin to relieve a cold or a pain? How many people do you know who take heavy doses of aspirin for rheumatoid arthritis and osteoarthritis? Yet is has been known since 1936 that aspirin interferes quite badly with vitamin C utilisation. If you take 600 mg of acetylsalicylic acid (that is two aspirins) every six hours, the result is a 100 per cent increase in the twenty-four hour urinary excretion of ascorbic acid. And 2,400 mg is not unusual in the daily treatment of arthritis. Yet, ironically, ascorbic acid actually *improves* the efficacy of aspirin by increasing its absorption, thereby accelerating pain relief, ensuring slower excretion and a longer lasting, all-round effect from the aspirin. Being a herbalist I don't approve of the use of aspirin, which levies a heavy tax on the adrenal glands and impairs the clotting function of platelets, and which I believe is actually harmful in the treatment of collagen illness like arthritis. There are alternative natural methods of coping with the pain and inflammation of arthritis (of which more in Chapter 10) and certainly it has been noticed that patients with this disease often have low levels of vitamin C in the blood (see a study in the *Lancet* of 8 May 1971 by Drs M. A. Sahud and R. J. Cohen). So it seems to me to be a sensible precaution to preserve a high level of ascorbic acid within the body by supplementing the diet with extra vitamin C.

Barbiturates, which happily are now giving way to safer drugs, tetracyclines and coricosteroids all affect the vitamin C status of the body in much the same way as aspirin. The lowered white blood cell level in turn results in a reduced ability to resist infection. You may not be too worried about the effects of these drugs, unless you are a chronic bronchitic or suffering from severe acne, for example, in which case you may be on treatment with tetracyclines for prolonged periods, but what about the pill? Recent studies of women taking the contraceptive pill, notably the oestrogenic one, have confirmed that their blood levels of vitamin C are consistently some thirty to forty per cent lower than those not on the pill. Bearing in mind that many of these women may be taking the contraceptive pill for thirty-five years without a break, surely nearly half a lifetime of reduced vitamin C status will have a very real effect on their general health? At the moment it is too soon to tell, but personally I'd rather they didn't wait for definitive proof. Similar considerations apply to women being treated with hormone replacement therapy.

Most people now know that every cigarette smoked destroys 25 mg of vitamin C, but if you give some thought to the cumulative consequences of this habit it may make you give up altogether. A packet of cigarettes daily reduces the ascorbic acid in the blood by forty per cent and this rises to a staggering fifty per cent in males smoking this number of cigarettes daily aged between forty and sixty-four. So twenty-a-day smokers must at least double their vitamin C intake to maintain the same levels as non-smokers. And for those non-smokers living with heavy smokers, it has been demonstrated that they inhale enough tobacco smoke to put their own vitamin C status at risk. Besides which non-smokers married to smokers have eighty per cent of their chances of developing lung cancer. An extremely sobering thought.

Alcohol also destroys vitamin C and even a moderate daily drinker should be aiming at an ascorbic acid intake of at least a gram a day. Chronic drinkers would do well to remember that one of the standard emergency treatments for alcoholics admitted to hopsital in a coma is an intravenous infusion of vitamin C, often accompanied by the B complex, particularly B_1. Tragically, the very vitamins and minerals needed to detoxify alcohol effectively are those influenced to the highest degree by alcohol and its converted poison acetaldehyde.

Generally vitamin C reserves in the body decrease as age increases, so the elderly are most at risk here, and men more so than women (although the specific reason for this anomaly is not yet known). Such people don't show the obvious signs of scurvy but manifest vitamin C deficiency in symptoms lower down the scale – depression, personality changes and many irritating non-specific minor illnesses. Sadly, it has been found that all those people who have to spend prolonged periods in institutions for whatever reason are most at risk in their vitamin C reserves, presumably because of poor dietary intake.

In view of all these considerations it seems that those of us experiencing some form of prolonged stress, drinkers, smokers, women on the pill, those taking prolonged courses of certain drugs and the elderly, particularly the institutionalised, need higher doses of vitamin C to maintain their correct body level. I've already stated that the government-recommended dose in this country is ludicrously low and would recommend a daily minimum dose of 1,000 mg and a much higher dose for all those exceptions up to 4,000 mg daily. A therapeutic dose can go as high as 20,000 mg daily but this must be taken under supervision.

What happens to vitamin C inside the body?

This is an important consideration because, not only is it water-soluble, and therefore continually flushed out of the body by urination, but the body can only cope with a certain level of intake at any one time. The gastro-intestinal tract is capable of absorbing up to eighty per cent of 250 mg of vitamin C ingested at one time into the bloodstream. But as the intake rises so the extent of absorption decreases. Only fifty per cent of a single dose of 2,000 mg can be absorbed, and 1,200 mg of a single 3,000 mg dose. The secret, therefore, to get round this, is to take in your vitamin C in small doses throughout the day.

However, if you are taking supplementation, this does not apply to the high-potency *prolonged*-release type of tablet. Such tablets are specifically manufactured to ensure they disintegrate very slowly on their journeys through the gut, releasing their vitamin C as they go, which ensures that the absorption of ascorbic acid is sustained. This is a man-made way of imitating what generally happens in nature when vitamin C-rich food is eaten, giving up its ascorbic acid content on its slow passage through the gut. In other words, the complex structure of food constituents leads to a built-in prolonged-release mechanism.

For those die-hards who are staggered at my high-dose suggestion of vitamin C let us consider its safety. By and large ascorbic acid is recognised as one of the safest of all vitamins, even when taken in massive doses, but its toxic effects include gastro-intestinal upsets such as nausea, cramps and diarrhoea, frequent urination (high doses certainly act as a diuretic), a corrosive effect on the mouth and teeth and skin rashes. I should emphasise that all these symptoms are very unusual and may be quickly reversed by lowering the dosage. Besides which they are easily and quickly noticed by the individual concerned before they get out of hand.

I would also advise that individuals who know they have kidney disease and people being treated with anticoagulent drugs seek the advice of an orthomolecular therapist before they start dosing themselves with any extra supplementation of vitamin C, nor should vitamin C ever be taken with ginseng.

Sources of vitamin C

The quantity of this vitamin present in plants varies widely among species and even among different samples of the same species, and much depends on the degree of ripeness and the source. It seems that climatic conditions are far more important than soil quality in determining the vitamin C content of oranges, the most familiar source of this vitamin. Orange trees grown on the coast invariably contain more vitamin C than those

grown inland. They are by no means the richest source of
vitamin C. The acerola cherry, which grows in the West Indies,
and the camu-camu plum, an Amazonian fruit, far outrank the
orange, as you can appreciate from the following table. Vitamin
C is usually measured in milligrams, although occasionally you
may see it expressed in units, in which case 1.0 mg equals 20
units. The following list shows the richest sources of vitamin C
in descending order when compared weight for weight.

Parsley	Chicory
Blackcurrants (fresh)	Radishes
Blackcurrants (stewed)	Peas
Broccoli	Limes
Green peppers	Melons
Tomato purée	Pineapples
Brussels sprouts	Raspberries
Chives	Swedes
Spearmint	Sweet potatoes
Savoy cabbage	Turnips
Watercress	Tomatoes
Strawberries	Runner beans
Red cabbage	Blackberries
Winter cabbage	Asparagus
Spinach	Avocado Pears
Oranges	Cooking apples
Orange juice	Lettuce
Mustard tops	Bananas
Redcurrants	Onions
Turnip tops	Cherries
White cabbage	Sweetcorn
Grapefruit	Rhubarb
Gooseberries	Eating apples
Mustard and cress	Peaches
New potatoes	Pears
Spring greens	Blueberries

Unusual sources of vitamin C

Acerola cherry and camu-camu plum are spectacularly high in
vitamin C. The following also contain reasonable amounts:

Rosehips	Wild strawberry leaves

Guavas
Violet leaves
Wintercress buds
Violet blossoms
Wintercress leaves
Dockleaves
Kale
Horseradish
Cranberries
Goosefoot
Green amaranth
Nettles

Catnip leaves
Ground ivy
Lychees
Loganberries
Dandelion leaves
Dandelion buds
Purslane
Bilberries
Prickly pears
Quinces
Elderberries

Other plants known to be rich in vitamin C but which have not yet been quantified include barberries, coltsfoot, sea buckthorn, coriander, garlic, knotgrass, plantain, nasturtium leaves, oregano, and chickweed. Seeds are also a useful form of vitamin C but only once they have been sprouted. On average they contain 9-15 mg of this vitamin per ounce. Sir Francis Chichester made sure he had a regular supply of vitamin C by growing mustard and cress on his epic solo voyage round the world.

Vitamin P (bioflavonoids)

The term 'vitamin P' is now technically redundant since the American Institute of Nutrition decided that 'bioflavonoid' is more appropriate as it covers a whole gamut of chemically related substances that have a common biological effect. Only a few of these have a distinct biochemical action, the others are clinically useless. The most potent belong to a class of methoxylated bioflavonoids which occur almost exclusively in the white pith of citrus fruits.

What are they for?

One of the most life-saving aspects of bioflavonoids could be their anti-thrombosis property. Blood contains a natural anti-thrombosis factor called heparin which is manufactured by the body. It has recently been discovered that, weight for weight, nobiletin (one of the bioflavonoids present in citrus fruits) is as active as heparin in its anti-thrombotic activity. But so far tests in this area have only been conducted on animals, not humans.

However, bioflavonoids have been successfully used to prevent habitual miscarriages, to arrest postnatal bleeding, nosebleeds, bleeding gums, menstrual disorders, haemorrhoids and widespread bruising. You will gather from this list that bioflavonoids are essential for the maintenance of healthy capillaries. Their specific anti-inflammatory action resides in nobiletin and another compound called tangeretin, both of which also stimulate body enzymes which in turn detoxify carcinogenic substances inside the body. Both have anti-bacterial and anti-viral properties.

Quercetin, myricetin and kaempferol play some part in preventing cataracts as well as acting as natural antioxidants. The best known bioflavonoid, rutin, is believed to be effective in the treatment of high blood pressure, arteriosclerosis and bruising.

How much?

All this would suggest that the whole wide spectrum of the active bioflavonoids need to be taken on a regular basis if they are to carry out their proper protective role in the body. Plants that are rich in these compounds are all the citrus fruits, especially lemons (remember they occur in the white pith, not the fruit itself), apricots, cherries, grapes, green peppers, tomatoes, broccoli, cabbage, plums, parsley, blackberries, blackcurrants and buckwheat. Interestingly, you will see from this list that wherever bioflavonoids occur in nature so does vitamin C. The two act as partners and, in illnesses which involve capillary fragility, one simply will not work unless accompanied by the other. This is another good argument for the use of natural as opposed to synthetic vitamins. As early as 1954 experiments showed that vitamin C and bioflavonoids administered together speed up the recovery from the common cold much more than synthetic vitamin C given alone. I feel the optimum dose of bioflavonoid is about 1,000 mg a day, though if you're ingesting the appropriate amount of vitamin C in its natural form this amount of bioflavonoid will inevitably accompany it. A therapeutic dose can go as high as 3,000 mg without any difficulty.

Vitamin D

This vitamin has, erroneously, been called 'the sunshine
vitamin' because many imagine it is contained in the sun's rays.
There are only two of the twenty different forms of this vitamin
which are of any practical use to the body, D_2 and D_3, and the
former is produced by the action of the sun's ultraviolet rays on
the surface of the skin.

What is it for?

The exact process is still not fully understood but what seems to
happen is this: the oil glands of the skin, when bathed in the
ultraviolet light of the sun or the light from a mercury-vapour
quartz lamp, secrete a wax like pro-vitamin called irradiated
7-dehydrocholesterol which in turn is believed to be converted
into vitamin D_2, then absorbed by the skin into the bloodstream.
So, when animals lick their coats, what they are actually doing is
ingesting vitamin D!

Vitamin D controls an enzyme called phosphatase which is
essential for bone formation. Without the vital help of vitamin D
bone growth is slowed down and the formation of healthy teeth
delayed. The long-term effects of such deprivation are irrepar-
able, because once the bones harden they remain in their
assumed formation for good or ill. If the latter, children will
develop bow legs, knock knees, curved spines and eventually
rickets.

Vitamin D also helps to release energy within the body.
Phosphorus carries blood sugar through the intestinal wall and
into the liver where it is converted into glycogen and stored.
Blood sugar is one of the necessary fuels for energy, and children
with low vitamin D stores burn less blood sugar and suffer from
lassitude. It has been suggested that children who have an
insatiable craving for sweets may actually be lacking vitamin D.
Those of us who spend most of the winter hibernating indoors,
well covered in clothes, may also suffer from lack of energy
during these months, and if you notice this pattern establishing
itself on a yearly basis, pay particularly attention to your vitamin
D intake and make sure you eat the foods rich in it from
September to April.

Vitamin D also plays an important part in the health of the

eyes. A shortage may result in myopia. One of the difficulties in detecting such a lack is the extreme vagueness of its symptoms – lack of energy, an insidious, creeping muscular weakness and stiffness. All of these are often accepted with resignation as the penalties of old age, which is particularly worrying as it is the elderly who are most likely to suffer from lack of vitamin D.

How many elderly people do you see sunbathing? How many regularly drink a daily pint of milk fortified with vitamin D? Sadly, with the swing in Western Europe towards the insular nuclear family, too many of them live lonely lives shut away indoors, supported by inadequate pensions and ignorant about their dietary needs. Osteomalacia in the elderly corresponds to rickets in children, and many doctors may well be treating as symptoms of old age what is in reality a deficiency. Knowing, as they do, that milk is now irradiated with vitamin D, they sometimes forget that many adults and children don't drink it, and others, in our cholesterol – and weight-conscious society, will only touch the fat-free variety which contains no vitamin D. Because cheese and fat are so high in calories they may cut these out altogether. So a deficiency in vitamin D is not so hard to come by.

Black and brown skin, or very deeply tanned skin, only allow three to thirty-six per cent of the ultraviolet rays from the sun through the outermost horny layer of the skin, while white skin lets in fifty-three to seventy-two per cent. It is as well to remember this, because in many parts of the Third World the effect sunlight has on the skin is still the only adequate source of vitamin D.

Vitamin D and water

If you bath before enjoying a swim on a cloudless sunny day you'll be washing off the oils that form 7-dehydrocholesterol so that your body will be unable to form vitamin D. Similarly, if you shower or bath after swimming the oils will be washed off before your body has had time to absorb this vitamin. The solution to this dilemma? Don't wash or bath in the hour or two before going swimming, and enjoy a short lie in the sun after you come out of the pool or the sea.

Babies, who are greatly in need of vitamin D from their earliest formative weeks, should be gently rubbed down with a pad soaked in olive oil after a fifteen-minute supervised break in the sun. Don't wash them with soap and water after a sunbath and remember– a newborn infant will have to have the eyes and feet protected from the sun, and the skin should initially be exposed only for a few minutes. Build up to the fifteen minutes gradually.

In a country where the sun is so rarely seen (I speak as a spoiled colonial who enjoyed a childhood in sunny East Africa where I wore little but a pair of shorts and a smile), it is reassuring to know there are other sources of vitamin D. D_3 is present in very small amounts in eggs, butter, milk and in large quantities in fish liver oil and, indeed, in infinitesimal quantities in almost every fresh food.

Liver contains 1-400 IUs per 100 gram serving, egg yolk 1-5 IUs per gram and milk about 100 IUs per litre. Sunflower seeds are the only significant plant source of vitamin D, but it is possible to irradiate yeast and fungi artificially to make a synthetic vitamin D. This commercial vitamin D is 400,000 times stronger than a tablespoon of cod liver oil when given in equal volume but has distinct disadvantages, as you will see when you read the section on dosage.

The quantity of vitamin D varies according to the season. It is higher in the milk of cows allowed to browse and feed on summer grass than in the milk of those poor tethered animals seen in the Middle East, which are shut up all day in a dark stable and fed on straw.

How much?

As with all the fat-soluble vitamins, vitamin D is absorbed by mineral oil, so *never* take mineral oil as a constipation cure. Apart from this consideration, mineral oil damages the liver. The absorption of vitamin D is also hindered by intestinal diseases such as coeliac syndrome, sprue and colitis. However, it is not sensitive to heat, light or oxygen.

Dosage is important because too much can be as harmful as too little, as this is one of the vitamins the body stores, mainly in the liver and blood, excreting it by way of the bile. If the body becomes overloaded with vitamin D and, in spite of its efforts, cannot get rid of any more through the bilary system, calcium metabolism is affected, leading to calcification of the bones, hardening of the arteries and mental retardation in children.

However, there is little cause for alarm if you take your vitamin D from natural sources. The possibility of getting addicted to cod liver oil or oily fish is pretty remote, and certainly in this country we don't see enough sun to make excess through conversion in the skin a danger. Even in clear weather, sunlight only contains an appreciable amount of ultraviolet light when it is thirty degrees from the horizon and this does not happen in the late autumn, winter and spring in our part of the world, which is nearly three-quarters of the year. Add to this industrial pollution, rain, dust and smog from our cities, ordinary window glass and clothing of even the lightest sort and you can see that we spend most of our lives excluding ultraviolet rays. But if you're a sun worshipper living in sunnier climes, remember vitamin B_1 has a protective action against any possible overdose of vitamin D.

Babies from birth to three weeks should have 350 IUs a day, graduating to 700 IUs in the second month. Teenagers should be drinking a quart of milk a day as well as 1,000 IUs as their need is very high. Adults should be taking between 500 to 1,000 IUs daily, and studies at the Henry Ford Hospital in Detroit indicate that an adult can take 4,000 IUs a day as part of the treatment for certain illnesses, but this should always be done under medical supervision. There is such a wide variation in the adult dosage because much depends on lifestyle. If you're a farmer working outdoors in all weathers, or a life-guard, you're going to need much less than an office worker or coal miner. Old people are advised to stick to the high end of the scale. To give you some idea about large doses, between 1,000-3,000 IUs will cure rickets and 10,000 IUs is a toxic dose.

Vitamin F (unsaturated fatty acids)

Having struggled with a weight problem for years, I still remember my astonishment when Adelle Davis introduced me to the idea that some people are overweight precisely because they don't get enough fat. I had long been indoctrinated to the contrary and, being an inveterate calorie counter, avoided butter, cream and oil like the plague. Yet one of fat's beneficial roles in the body is the maintenance of the membrane walls that enclose all living cells. If the membrane is damaged or caves in, the contents of the cell seep out. As most of it is liquid (our bodies are sixty per cent water) some people who look fat are simply swollen and waterlogged. More importantly, when overweight people cut out fats, their bodies change sugar to fat much more rapidly than normal in an effort to produce missing nutrients. This makes blood sugar drop quickly, which in turn makes them ragingly hungry, so they overeat. It is now an established fact that fats are far more sustaining than sugary or starchy foods, so it is essential to include a little with every meal, to keep you from the biscuit tin in between as your blood sugar plunges.

Apart from membrane walls round the thyroid, kidneys, skin and nerve sheaths all rely on fat for healthy maintenance. Fat marries up with oxygen to produce energy, and with cholesterol to form a combined fatty substance that goes on to be broken down and used for growth, energy and skin health. It is essential to ensure the efficient production of bile (too little may lead to gall-stones) and the fat-splitting enzyme lipase. Fatty acids cooperate with vitamin D in its effort to make calcium available to the body, and they do this by helping in the assimilation of phosphorus and by nourishing the skin.

A deficiency in the fatty acids is very easy to spot – frequent stubborn colds, dry skin (including infantile and adult eczema and dandruff), hair and nails becoming brittle and dull, diarrhoeal conditions, boils and acne, varicose ulcers, kidney disease or thyroid disorder.

What kind of fat?

Don't make the mistake of lumping all fats under one heading. The three unsaturated fatty acids that your body is unable to produce are linoleic acid, linolenic acid and arachidonic acid. All of these are found in cereal and vegetable fats and oils – wheatgerm, safflower, cotton, rye-germ, maize-germ, sunflower, soya bean, peanut, linseed, palm and olive oils. But there is very little present in margarine, hydrogenated cooking fats, or the animal fats such as butter, cream, beef or mutton or fish oil.

To ensure that you are getting your fatty acids read the label. It must say 'dehydrogenated' which means, essentially, the way that fat is produced in nature (see page 23). Do not be misled by the words 'cold-pressed' which is rapidly becoming as flagrantly misused as 'natural' is with cosmetics. A good unrefined oil will taste and smell aromatically nutty. Sesame and olive oils are the most stable, but all oils should be kept cool in a pantry or fridge. Don't be hoodwinked by a label which says 'rich in polyunsaturates', because this also indicates it has been processed and as a result its nutritional value has been drastically reduced.

This is yet another example of the wisdom of nature, for wherever vitamin F occurs in plants it is always accompanied by vitamin E – an essential partnership, because vitamin E prevents vitamin F from combining with oxygen in the air and becoming rancid. Most of the vitamin E present in cereals is found in the germ of the grain, which is usually discarded when the germ is processed to produce oil. As the vitamin F is left unprocessed, the oil is liable to spoil and go rancid quickly, mainly due to the linoleic acid. So food processors ensure a longer shelf life by extracting the linoleic acid and adding an antioxidant. When you eat this preserved oil the body is unable to separate the remaining fractions of vitamin F from the antioxidant, so the oil is, in effect, useless and cannot do its allotted task. It is simply stored as fat or discarded. So you can see how important it is to scrutinise the label.

The body is quite capable of converting sugar to fats, but remember it cannot manufacture unsaturated fatty acids, so you must ensure an adequate supply by using a tablespoon of the cold-pressed oils daily in salad dressings or by eating at least two ounces of whole grains and seeds. Don't eat processed fats if you can avoid them. They're only good for putting on weight. Above all don't eat rancid fats of any kind, because these destroy vitamins A, D, E and K in the food itself or in the intestine. You may think there's not much danger of that because your taste buds would soon shout a warning, but you'd be surprised how often cake mixes, pastry mixes, potato crisps, popcorn and salted nuts are held too long in storage and as a result are rancid. A touch of rancidity is often masked by the more powerful flavours of salt or sugar. Keep your cold-pressed oils in the fridge to ensure they don't go off.

Vitamin K

What is it for?
Vitamin K is essential for the synthesis by the liver of the blood clotting enzyme prothrombin, without which we'd bleed to death. The intestinal bacteria in our bodies are capable of producing vitamin K in appropriate quantities regardless of how

much we ingest from food, and you may think that this being the case you have no problems. True, provided you're perfectly healthy, but consider the following exceptions. If you have jaundice, gall-stones, inadequate bile production in the liver, damaged intestines (as a result of, say, severe diarrhoea or colitis), a damaged liver or if you're on a course of antibiotics, then vitamin K cannot be either properly absorbed or synthesised.

Vitamin K works well with vitamin C to fend off morning sickness, the ideal combination being 5 mg of K and 23 mg of C taken together daily. As is true of the cooperation between so many other vitamins, one will not work in this area without the other. Vitamin K is particularly helpful whenever anticoagulant drugs are being taken for heart conditions to stop clots forming in the blood, and people who are the victims of heart problems must make certain they are eating plenty of vitamin K.

Perhaps its most interesting use is for the control of pain. The Yugoslavians have discovered that this vitamin has a more calming effect than morphine in many patients suffering from terminal cancers. The dose used in the experiment to ascertain this was up to 30 mg.

It has also been discovered that older people, those beyond the age of fifty-six, who are seriously diseased have a much lower than normal ability to coagulate blood and all will benefit from extra vitamin K, providing the intestine is not so badly damaged it is unable to absorb it.

How much?

The minimum daily requirement to ensure blood clotting is 0.03 mg of vitamin K to every kilogram of body weight, so you can work out your own requirement.

Sources

Luckily, the plant world abounds in vitamin K. It is present in alfalfa, all dark green leafy plants especially spinach, cauliflower, cabbage, carrot tops, kale, soya beans and soya bean oil, seaweed and pine needles. It is most concentrated in the greenest parts of the plant. There are some traces of it in animal sources like egg yolk, but by comparison with plants the quantities present are minute.

Vitamin K is available in synthetic form but it can be highly toxic in large doses, so once again I would champion the superiority of natural sources, for you'd find it awfully hard to gorge on enough spinach to poison yourself with this particular vitamin.

As well as being destroyed by antibiotics, vitamin K is also vulnerable in the presence of aspirins and the other salicylates and is sensitive to light, air, oxygen, strong acids and alcoholic alkalis. So eat your green leafy plants raw, prepare them at the last minute to ensure maximum freshness and go easy on the lemon juice.

Vitamin E

Before 1912 cardiovascular disease was virtually unknown, yet today Britain ranks first in the world as far as heart problems are concerned. Why? Partly because of our increasingly sedentary lives, environmental pollution and the vast array of chemicals we now eat. But an even more significant factor is the leaching of vitamin E from our food. Modern flour processing, using steel-roller milling, removes eighty-seven per cent of the seven vitamins present in wheat, eighty-four per cent of bulk minerals and eighty-eight per cent of trace metals. This bleached flour is then 'enriched' with a smattering of some of the vitamins that have so painstakingly been removed – B_1, B_2, B_5. Ferrous sulphate is then finally added in sufficient quantity to neutralise any last lingering traces of vitamin E. Processed breakfast cereals made from maize, oats, rice and wheat are leached of nearly ninety per cent of their vitamin E, as is hydrogenated oil and margarine. So if we're lucky we finish up ingesting 5-8 IUs of this vitamin daily, the minimum quantity the FDA recommend for babies.

What is it for?
Firstly, it reduces the need of the tissue cells for oxygen. Living in a world polluted by chemicals and smokers, our bodies have constantly to fight off the destructive oxidising impact on the delicate membranes of our lungs. Vitamin E helps, and I have given it to patients suffering from the sort of emotional and physical strains which lead to breathing problems, like asthma, with some success.

Secondly, vitamin E helps to melt blood clots, prevent thrombosis, expand blood vessels and capillaries and strengthen their walls, opening up new channels of blood supply where others are blocked and so improving circulation to a 'half dead' area – such as coronary occlusion. By dilating capillaries which bring blood and oxygen right up to the surface of the skin, it helps the treatment of burns, wounds, chronic ulcers and some types of skin disease. Because of all these beneficial actions on the vascular system it impedes the formation of internal and external scar tissue.

It is essential for the normal blood clotting process, multiplying the number of healthy platelets in the bloodstream. In a quarter of those diabetic types who suffer with circulation problems which may result in gangrene, it reduces the need for insulin. It is also one of the vitamins used to excellent effect in megadoses of 800 IUs in the treatment of hypoglycaemia. It acts as a safe diuretic because it does not leach minerals from the body in the process. Indeed, one of its most important functions is to protect other essential nutrients, vitamin A, C, F and the sulphur-containing amino acids both in the body and in food containing these elements. Being a herbalist, I naturally do not approve of the long-term use of analgesics, and for those unfortunate patients who've been eating aspirins like smarties for years to treat arthritis, I wean them off while gradually introducing vitamin E to protect against their harmful side-effects. Vitamin E also neutralises the harmful effect of large doses of paracetamol, useful in cases of parasuicide.

It normalises the activity of ovaries in women, improving and preventing problems like dysmenorrhoea and menopausal problems. (For dryness and irritation of the vagina it needs to be administered in suppository form.) It is helpful in the treatment of chronic cystic mastitis. Women on the pill are in special need of vitamin E because oestrogen in the pill can lead to blood clots and phlebitis, and it protects against these. It also improves the number and quality of sperm cells in semen. Finally, because it regulates the metabolism of fats and proteins, it has a profound effect on all the body's processes.

Deficiencies of this vitamin are not hard to come by. The persistent inability to absorb fats, through all sorts of lingering intestinal illnesses leads to reduced absorption of vitamin E and can be remedied by megadoses of the *water-solubilised* form.

People who've had heart attacks are often placed on diets which are high in polyunsaturated fats while saturated animal fats are radically reduced. In such cases it is essential to bear in mind that polyunsaturated fats cut down the body's vitamin E supply and actually create a deficiency by internal attrition, so vitamin E intake should be commensurate with the amount of polyunsaturated fat in the diet, 0.6 IUs per gram of polyunsaturated fat. Mineral oil blocks the absorption of vitamin E and anyway is no way to cope with constipation.

Irritable babies with haemolytic anaemia and oedema may well be vitamin E deficient, but in adults the signs are much harder to detect. They may be as vague as apathy, lethargy, lack of concentration, muscular weakness, irritability and worsening sexual performance. A true deficiency really needs to be checked by laboratory tests when other factors like increased fragility of red blood cells and increased creatine in the urine will be taken into account.

How much?

The recommended daily dose, which is 5 IUs for babies to 30 IUs for adults, does not take into account the losses during food processing and how much of this vitamin the body can actually absorb in individual cases, remembering that a mild deficiency (which is what most people suffer from) can eventually build up to a gross one. Women in the menopause need ten times more vitamin E than normal and, as one enters old age, that need increases to more than fifty times the ordinary inadequate dose which is normally about 10 IUs.

I advise a normal supplementary dose of somewhere between 400 and 800 IUs taken just after meals to ensure maximum utilisation. Very high therapeutic doses can go up to 6,000 IUs and I have heard of the dosage in the treatment of Crohn's disease reaching 16,000 IUs but of course this must be done under medical supervision.

Because vitamin E influences the body's processes so widely, I think it is always wise to start with a low level of 100 IUs daily for a month, and then build up to 200 IUs in the following month and so on until the individually required dose is reached. You can pause and persevere at any level, whether it is for a passing problem like menopausal complaints, or for a chronic illness like diabetes. A word of caution: people with uncontrolled hypertension, overactive thyroids, diabetes and chronic rheumatic heart disease *must* be treated under medical supervision. Failure to observe this stricture will result in some very unpleasant side-effects. Otherwise vitamin E is perfectly safe when used in the normal doses I have specified. Symptoms of vitamin E excess are similar to those I have already listed for its deficiency, and a simple reduction of the dose to a level where these symptoms are not produced indicates the amount of vitamin E an individual body can tolerate. If, for some reason, you're decreasing your dose of vitamin E, do so gently and gradually.

Sources

Vitamin E is made up of four tocopherols, the most important being alpha-tocopherols. If the vitamin is being taken as a supplement, the d-alpha-tocopherol is the preferred type. Its richest source is cereal grains and their oils, green leaves and seeds, but the tocopherol level of the extracted oils are of course influenced by the source of the plant, its harvesting time, storage and processing conditions. Best to read the labels and buy genuinely cold-pressed virgin oils, expressed by the hydraulic process method, which are not leached of their vitamin E content, and to store them well-sealed in a cool pantry. Vitamin E is sensitive to alkaloids, oxygen and ultraviolet light, so wheatgerm should be stored in a sealed container in the fridge. There are traces of vitamin E in lettuce, tomatoes, parsley, carrots, egg yolk, fish roe and nuts, but not enough to get excited about. This means that vitamin E really needs to be taken in its cold-pressed oil or its fresh cereal form. Cooking does not destroy it substantially (it loses about eleven per cent when heated for frying).

The following oils are richest in vitamin E oil in descending order:

Extra virgin olive	Cottonseed
Sunflower	Safflower
Grapeseed	Coconut
Wheatgerm	Peanut
Ricebran	Rapeseed

Be careful with cottonseed oil. The Chinese have discovered that in large doses it causes liver cancer.

CHAPTER 3

Minerals

Vitamins have excited scientific imagination since the 1980s to such a degree that it is now seldom appreciated that, without the subtle help of minerals, vitamins are absolutely useless. But if you're taking your vitamins in their natural form in food don't worry – once again nature has achieved perfect balance. Wherever there is a vitamin-rich herb there are also large quantities of minerals present.

Every nutrient in the body, proteins, enzymes, amino acids, and carbohydrates – not just vitamins – needs minerals in order to make it work. But minerals go further than this: they also have a sparing action on vitamins and protein, meaning that less of these items are necessary in the diet if minerals are particularly abundant. But, as with vitamins, no mineral works in isolation.

For ease of reference I have placed the minerals in alphabetical order.

Bromine

This little-known mineral is directly influenced by the pituitary gland and is contained in the blood. When the level of bromine drops it is now known to lead to certain types of depression, notably PMT and menopausal blues. Foods rich in bromine are all the melon family, cucumber, celery, apples, garlic, peaches, asparagus, tomatoes and lettuce.

Calcium

Calcium is an excellent example of the essential link between minerals and vitamins. It must have vitamin A, C and D as well as phosphorus in order to function. Our bodies have more calcium than any other mineral, and ninety per cent of it is in our bones and teeth. The rest circulates in the body fluids and helps the metabolic processes, particularly that of digestion, as well as the proper working of the parathyroid gland. A deficiency leads to osteoporosis (brittle bones) and an adult version of rickets, acidosis, insomnia, irritability and the improper healing of wounds. Adelle Davis describes calcium as being as soothing as a mother, as relaxing as a sedative and as life-giving as an oxygen tent. A good dose of calcium is 800 mg but you can go as high as 3000 mg, and high doses are particularly necessary in the growing years as well as during pregnancy and while breastfeeding.

It is richly present in kelp, Irish moss, dulse, nettles, turnip tops, mustard, parsley and is also available in camomile flowers and the leaves of chicory, cleavers, coltsfoot, dandelion, horsetail, meadowsweet, mistletoe, pimpernel, plantain, purslane, rest-harrow, shepherd's purse, silverweed, sorrel, toadflax, watercress, willow, yellow dock and the young shoots of poke weed.

It is one of the two minerals – the other being iron – that needs hydrochloric acid for assimilation. If your stomach is not producing enough, sip a little diluted cider vinegar before taking your calcium. It is not affected by light or heat.

Chlorine

Coupled with sodium, this mineral maintains the balance between fluids inside and outside the body's cells, ensuring osmotic equilibrium so that muscles and nerves contract appropriately, blood coagulates and wounds heal. It has been likened to nature's broomstick because it sweeps poisons out of the system, stimulating the liver, inducing the proper production of hydrochloric acid in the stomach, and efficiently distributing the hormones secreted by the endocrine glands. It maintains suppleness of joints and tendons and stops the overformation of fatty tissue.

Large quantities of chlorine exist as chlorides in almost all foods and it is *not* necessary to take sodium chloride, common table salt, in order to get a sufficient quantity of this mineral. All the grasses, nettles and comfrey are especially rich in chlorine, as are blackberries and raspberries, and it is also available in parsley, horseradish, watercress, dandelions, lettuce, chicory, spinach and turnip tops.

Chromium

This plays a vital role in the way the liver synthesises fatty acids and cholesterol, the way the pancreas controls blood sugar levels and enzyme activation. Adequate amounts are vital to ensure a normal glucose utilisation and proper fat metabolism, and are very important for hyper- and hypo-glycaemics. Unsaturated fats, bone meal, mushrooms, molasses and whole grains are rich in chromium. Brewer's yeast is a particularly good source of this mineral.

Copper

Copper is needed to convert the body's iron into haemoglobin and it very rapidly floods into the bloodstream after ingestion. It is also necessary for the formation of elastin throughout the body, for the proper development of bones, brain, nerves and enzyme function. Our problem nowadays tends to be too much rather than too little, and high levels of copper are toxic, accumulating in the blood and depleting the brain's zinc supply and leading to arteriosclerosis, high blood pressure, and kidney diseases connected with ageing. If you've got copper water pipes in the house you'll be unwittingly ingesting copper, particularly if you tend to fill up the kettle from the hot tap or if you live in a soft water area. In this case use a water purifier. Other sources include the pill, copper cooking utensils, the copper IUD, some vitamin-mineral supplements which also contain copper, raisins, and shell fish which live in copper-rich waters. A high copper intake tends to depress zinc levels in the body.

A copper deficiency is extremely rare, and if it happens generally does so because of a diet heavily dependent on refined foods and whole milk. Shellfish, especially oysters, offal, wheat, dried fruit, almonds and beans are rich sources of copper. A daily dose really shouldn't go above 1-2 mg.

Fluorine

By this I mean *natural* fluorine. The type added to drinking water, sodium fluoride, is a by-product of some fifty different types of industry, including the steel, aluminium and phosphate fertiliser industries. Off-putting? Well, I'll go further and say synthetic fluoride is poisonous, it inhibits the function of vitamin C and in excess weakens bones and mottles the enamel on teeth.

The fluoride found in nature, calcium fluoride, is not dangerous. Quite the opposite – it acts as an anti-infective, maintaining the health of the entire body including the eyes. It is present in naturally fluoridated water, beet leaves, garlic and watercress.

Iodine

Iodine is vital to the health of the thyroid gland and, when examining a patient's iris (one of the diagnostic tools I use), I rarely see a perfectly healthy thyroid. This is particularly true of people over forty. An American Medical Association report published some years ago concluded that fifty-five per cent of women and forty-five per cent of men who believed themselves to be healthy were low in thyroid activity, and I believe the figures are escalating. Of the 25 mg present in blood and tissues, 15 mg resides in the thyroid, stimulating it to secrete a hormone called thyroxin that regulates metabolism and energy. A deficiency can lead to goitre, anaemia, listlessness, slow pulse, low blood pressure, obesity, increasing irritability and dry hair that easily breaks. Those of us who live more than 100 miles from the sea are eating vegetables grown in soil which lacks iodine, and it is here that kelp really comes into its own, for it will balance both under- and over-active thyroids. Together with dulse, laver and Irish moss, it is enormously rich in iodine, 1.5 per cent of its weight being organic iodine.

Those in need of added iodine, which is almost all of us, would do well to sprinkle a teaspoon of kelp powder daily over food and throw the salt cellar out of the window. A daily dose is 0.15 mg but one can go as high as 3 mg if in need of special help. Oestrogen is antagonistic to the proper functioning of the thyroid, so women on the pill are well advised to look to more organic iodine in their diets as well as vitamin E. People with underactive thyroids should skirt round cabbage and the rest of the brassica family, for large quantities aggravate iodine deficiency.

Iron

This works in harness with calcium and is essential to make the oxygen-carrying haemoglobin in red blood cells, thereby maintaining disease resistance, feeding nerve tissues and helping hair growth as well as assisting the enzyme reactions necessary for producing energy.

Lack of iron can lead to fuzzy memory, exhaustion, headaches, lethargy, sore cracks around the mouth, deformation of nails with ridging and brittleness, shortness of breath after exercise and finally anaemia.

Iron should *always* be taken in its natural form in food and herbs and it is most obviously present in herbs with very dark green leaves. The inorganic iron salts used in the 'enrichment' of food are known to lead to chronic disability and fatal disease in some people, notably children. Besides which, natural sources of iron are much better assimilated in the body and in turn help with the assimilation of vitamins C and E. Natural iron burns up accumulated poisonous wastes and flushes them out of the body, and unlike synthetic iron it does *not* cause constipation. Coffee or products with caffeine in them, like chocolate, inhibit iron absorption. A healthy stomach excreting sufficient hydrochloric acid is essential for its proper ingestion. A simple way to ensure this is to sip a teaspoon of cider vinegar diluted in water half an hour before each meal.

Iron is richly present in rice polishings, kelp, wheatgerm, sunflower seeds, parsley and apricots, as well as in purslane, the tops of beets and turnips, bilberry, blackberry, booklime, burdock, chicory, comfrey, cornflower, dandelion, yellow dock, gentian, groundsel, ground ivy, hawthorn, hops, nettles, periwinkle, raspberry, rest-harrow, rose, salep, scabious, scullcap, strawberries, toadflax, vervain, watercress, wood-sage, and wormwood.

Women use 15-30 mg of iron with each period and as much as 500 mg during childbirth. Children need more iron during their growing years, as do pregnant women and people suffering from blood loss, whether it be through bleeding piles, a stomach ulcer or ulceration in the intestines. Most people can manage on 20 mg daily but a high dose can go up to 120 mg.

Magnesium

Most of us are deficient in this mineral which, like calcium, displaces the strontium-90 present in radioactive fall-out. It works in harness with phosphorus and regulates the central nervous system, acts as an enzyme activator and promotes healthy glandular function. It is especially useful in the treatment of neuro-muscular problems – nervousness, tremors, tantrums, rages, oversensitivity to noise and epilepsy. It is an antacid and should be taken *before* meals to avoid clashing with calcium which needs acid for its proper assimilation. Another point to watch is that fluorides are strongly attracted to magnesium and, once linked, trap the magnesium in the body cells making it much less effective, another very good reason for avoiding water with sodium fluoride artificially added to it.

Lack of magnesium begins with chronic irritability and exhaustion and may finish with mental retardation and mental illness characterised by convulsions. Magnesium is abundantly present in soybeans, cashews, almonds and Brazil nuts and also available in alder, birch, broom, the tops of young carrots and beets, cowslips, dandelion, dulse, hops, kelp, marshmallow, meadow sweet, mistletoe, mullein, oak, oats, poppy, primrose, parsley, orchid, scabious, slippery elm, raspberry, rest-harrow, rose, toadflax, walnut leaves, watercress and spinach.

A daily dose should range from 100-400 mg but for therapeutic purposes one can go as high as 1,500 mg. The only people who need to tread carefully with magnesium are those with a kidney malfunction and they should take not more than 300 mg daily.

Manganese

Diabetics and those suffering from pancreatic disturbance, like hypoglycaemia, are generally deficient in this mineral and it is now believed that its lack may play a part in multiple sclerosis and myasthenia gravis. It works with the whole of the B group of vitamins to prevent sterility, is an important factor in the production of thyroxin, so helping the thyroid function properly, it helps the central nervous system to function normally and is needed for good enzymatic function so that food can be properly digested and utilised. Too much calcium and phosphorus blocks its absorption.

Manganese deficiency is hard to detect, but those with the diseases I've already mentioned, together with people with sluggish thyroids, those who suffer from recurrent dizziness, absent-mindedness and irritability would do well to boost their manganese intake. Normal doses range from 1-10 mg but you can go as high as 300 mg for short periods of time, as prolonged high doses will inhibit iron absorption. Manganese is richly present in nuts, all dark green leafy vegetables, peas, beetroot, blueberries, egg yolks, sunflower seeds, pineapple, kelp, whole grains.

When I had a spectrophotometry test done to determine the mineral levels in my body, no manganese showed up at all. Manganese deficiency is liable to become a widespread problem because of the way we farm, using lime and artificial fertilisation and so stopping plants absorbing it from the soil. I already knew from studying photographs of my eyes that my thyroid needed help, and realised I could support it better by boosting my manganese intake. (Manganese levels respond so slowly that a low level almost invariably necessitates supplementation.)

Phosphorus

Phosphorus often occurs with calcium and should be ingested in the ratio of 2½ parts of calcium to one of phosphorus, because whenever it is excreted it drags an even bigger proportion of calcium with it. Phosphorus is second only to calcium as far as bones and teeth are concerned, it has a tonic effect on the circulation and is essential for muscle action, nerve coordination, fat and starch metabolism, enzyme formation and the sparking of energy. Some cases of obesity can be traced to its lack, as can general fatigue, nervous disorders, poor resistance to infection and mental apathy. White sugar badly disrupts the delicate calcium/phosphorus balance. A daily dose can be as high as 1000 mg, but always in its correct ratio to calcium.

Phosphorus is richly present in rice polishings, wheatgerm, sesame and sunflower seeds, dulse, kelp, Irish moss, parsley, watercress, as well as in anise, calamus, chickweed, cornflowers, dill, fenugreek, golden rod leaves, linseed, liquorice, marigold flowers and leaves, meadow-sweet flowers, sea holly, sweet flag flowers, sorrel, mustard, yellow dock, chicory, purslane, dandelion leaves and elderberries.

Potassium

While most of the sodium in the body is found outside the cells, potassium is found inside the same cells, and so they perform their delicate balancing act in perfect harmony, normalising the heartbeat, feeding the muscular system, balancing the body's water content and helping the kidneys to flush out waste, and feeding the bloodstream so the body's diseased tissue can heal quickly. Potassium alkalises the system, which is why I urge my arthritic and rheumatic patients to eat natural foods rich in it, knowing these foods contain the ideal potassium/sodium ratio so that uric acid is flushed away from painful joints. The process can be quite a vigorous one, so persistence is vital.

Deficiencies of potassium which especially afflict the elderly lead to muscular weakness, constipation, insomnia, problems with heartbeat, occasionally enlarged kidneys and brittle bones, or simply a general vague sense of unwellness.

Happily, potassium is abundant in most herbs and is especially rich in dulse, kelp, Irish moss, parsley, sunflower seeds, wheatgerm, as well as in the leaves of birch, borage, calamus, the top leaves of carrots, coltsfoot, comfrey, couch-grass, dandelion leaves, fennel, lady's mantle, meadow-sweet, mistletoe, mullein, mustard, nettle, oak, peony, peppermint, plantain, scullcap, shepherd's purse, sweetflag, toadflax, walnut leaves, wintergreen and wormwood, and the flowers of cowslip, camomile and primrose.

Silicon

Silicon works in the body to ensure calcium is properly used and not deposited where it is particularly unwelcome as nodes and spurs round joints. So those prone to arthritis are particularly in need of silicon. It works synergistically with calcium to strengthen hair and nails, and ensures effective elimination of toxins through the skin, as well as acting as insulation and protection to the nerve fibres.

A deficiency may lead to 'flabbiness' of the skin, chronic

fatigue, and I believe it is a contributory factor in arthritis. It is richly present in asparagus and strawberries and the leaves of bedstraw, cleavers, dandelion, flax, holly, horsetail, sea-holly, thistle, the stalks of all grasses and cereals, including wheat and oat, and in oats themselves, providing they are steel-cut rather than rolled. I always prescribe oatstraw and horsetail tea to my pregnant patients to ensure they're ingesting all the silicon they need, and if they moan about the taste I offer an alternative– two tablespoons of steel-cut oats soaked in purified warm water overnight, the water to be strained and drunk the next morning.

Sodium

This mineral works in harness with potassium, and together they control most of the fluid interacting within the body. Lack of sodium leads to excessive urination and eventually dehydration, to much severe oedema, hypertension, and I believe it is one of the contributory factors leading to arthritis. Sodium is the main alkaliser of the body, strengthening the digestive juices and sweetening the digestive tract. The kidneys become distressed if the sodium/potassium ratio is incorrect. Sodium stops catarrh and infections of the mucous membranes, and a sea salt and purified water snuff is the only way I let my patients take sodium chloride internally. It takes a little practice learning to snuff up this mixture correctly, a generous pinch to a cup of warmed purified water, but it works wonders, cleansing and strengthening the mucous membranes.

Luckily, nature in her wisdom has the sodium/potassium ratio perfectly balanced in all herbs – one part of sodium to five of potassium. It is richly present in all the sea plants, kelp, Irish moss, dulse, in the flowers and leaves of clover and violet, as well as in the leaves of alder, cleavers, comfrey, dandelion, dill, fennel, garlic, marshmallow, marguerite, meadow-sweet, mistletoe, mustard, nettles, parsley, rest-harrow, shepherd's purse, woodruff and watercress.

Every grain of salt retains 70 g of water in the body, so sodium chloride should never be added to the diet from the salt cellar. We need only 4 g daily and this is naturally present in the *natural* foods we eat. I stress natural, because as soon as you start into processed food your salt intake rockets. Try eating the conventional breakfast of cornflakes, which have considerable quantities of added salt, bacon and eggs, followed by marmite on toast, and your intake will have soared to 1500 mg from that meal alone. Most people in fact eat 20 g of sodium daily and it is now believed that over 14 g daily can produce toxic side-effects.

Sulphur

This purifies the whole system, particularly the blood, which is in turn responsible, among other things, for the health of the skin and hair, so not surprisingly it keeps the skin smooth, fingernails strong and the hair glossy. It also strengthens the glandular system, helps the flow of bile by keeping the liver healthy, and maintains the oxygen balance which is vital for proper brain function. Most of the body's sulphur comes from vitamin B, biotin and the amino acids which build tissues. Insulin is a sulphur compound, so diabetics really ought to eat food rich in sulphur, and as this is present in most protein, a wide variety of vegetables and herbs, this shouldn't be difficult. For the same reason a deficiency in sulphur is unknown.

One of the herbs richest in sulphur is garlic, which is a superb anti-infective. It is also present in marigold petals and in the leaves of brooklime, broom, calamus, chevril, coltsfoot, cowslip, daisy, dill, eyebright, fennel, Irish moss, marigold, meadow-sweet, mullein, nettles, nasturtium leaves, pimpernel, plaintain, poppy, primrose, rest-harrow, sage, scabious, sesame seeds, shepherd's purse, sweet flag, thyme and watercress.

Zinc

Zinc is manufactured in the pancreas, but then spreads out to almost every other area of the body, hair, all parts of the nervous system, skin, liver, bones, blood, kidneys, pituitary and male reproductive fluid. It helps to normalise the prostate, and insulin depends on zinc to function properly. It helps to utilise carbohydrates, heal wounds quickly, and protects against lead and some kinds of drug poisoning, particularly copper, and against TB. It also ensures that the heart and muscles work properly.

A deficiency is now believed to be a factor in schizophrenia, as well as leading to fatigue, susceptibility to infection and injury, arteriosclerosis, diarrhoea, stretch marks, irregular periods, poor circulation, white spots under the fingernails and dandruff. Excessive coffee intake and elevated levels of copper, calcium or cadmium aggravate low zinc levels.

Foods rich in zinc include brewer's yeast, seeds (especially pumpkin and sunflower seeds), green leafy vegetables, and above all liver. A daily dose should be 10 mg but one can go as high as 300 mg.

Toxic minerals

Lead, mercury, aluminium and cadmium are all toxic minerals which are becoming increasing menaces in our industrial society. The body doesn't need them in any shape or form and prolonged exposure to them decreases vitality, shortens the life, and generally aggravates disease. Exhaust fumes are the main source of lead, followed by lead piping and the solder used on food cans, cigarette smoke and lead-based pottery and glazes.

There's a growing body of evidence to suggest that increased body burdens of lead lowers IQ, decreases mental concentration, increases the rate of miscarriage, birth defects and still births, can lead to criminal and delinquent behaviour in children, increases the chances of getting cancer and generally speeds up the ageing process.

Mercury is present on the fungicides used to protect grain, in fish in mercury-saturated seas, some fabric softeners and floor waxes, mercury vapour lamps, some cosmetics, adhesives and dental amalgams. Like lead, mercury will cross the placental barrier during pregnancy, so that pregnant women exposed to it, though showing no signs of mercury poisoning themselves, may produce babies which are grossly mentally and physically deformed.

Smokers are known to have much higher levels of cadmium in their livers than non-smokers, and it is also present in tapwater from galvanised or plastic water pipes, tin cans, instant coffee, many processed meats, cola drinks and refined cereals which have a low zinc to cadmium range. Some scientists believe that cadmium is an even greater threat to health than either lead or mercury. Cadmium poisoning may result in hypertension, possibly emphysema, arteriosclerosis, cerebral haemorrhage, kidney and liver damage and eventually a painful softening of the bones.

Unlike lead and mercury, it is very hard to hustle cadmium out of the body quickly, but cadmium antagonists are calcium, iron, protein, vitamin D and zinc. So the way to protect oneself against toxicity would seem to be a diet rich in unprocessed foods and a reasonable degree of sunshine in an unpolluted atmosphere.

Aluminium in the form of aluminium cookware, aluminium foil, aluminated salt (which includes most table salt), baking powder, antacids, toothpaste, cigarette filters, buffered aspirin, cosmetics, hot water heaters with aluminium cathodes, processed cheese, cosmetics and pharmaceuticals is ubiquitously with us. Toxic symptoms begin with persistent indigestion and lead on to gastrointestinal upset, rickets (by interfering with phosphate absorption), psoriasis, cystic fibrosis and senility. Aluminium is highly reactive to alkaline saliva, so that by the time food cooked in aluminium saucepans hits your stomach, gas is being produced in just the same way as baking powder acts as a cake rises. To some extent the hydrochloric acid in the stomach keeps this under control, but the real problem begins in the duodenum. So cook in iron, earthenware, china, glass, stainless steel, or, as I do, in enamel-lined saucepans but **never** cook or bake in aluminium. The aluminium in the food ingested from the saucepans will then go on reacting and producing painful gas all the way through to the colon, adding insult to injury by upsetting the delicate pH of the whole digestive tract, flooding the bloodstream and burdening the body's organs. Aluminium is cumulative, so the overall effect gets worse as we get older. The good news is that aluminium can be sped out of the body by eating foods high in pectin, particularly bananas, apples, lemons, lemon rind and sunflower seeds.

If you're worried about the mineral content in your body, believing it may be distorted or inadequate, you can get a mineral analysis of your hair done by a reputable laboratory in California. (The address is in the appendix.) Unfortunately there is no equivalent facility here as yet, but I gather 'Foresight', a charitable association for preconceptual care, is working on it. If you want to begin by detoxifying yourself, before embarking on a programme to rebalance your minerals (and as almost every one of us has too much lead, aluminium and mercury in our system it may not be a bad idea), start like this:

Heavy mineral three month detoxifying programme

Take the following items every day for 3 months:

1. 2 level teaspoons of kelp powder or 2 sheets of dulse, nori seaweed or laver.
2. 1 cup of home-made apple sauce. Cook the apples with a squeeze of lemon juice and plenty of grated lemon rind. During digestion the apple pectin is transformed into galateuric acid, which combines with the toxic metals to form an insoluble metallic salt, which is then excreted. The best utilised source of pectin as far as the body is concerned is home-made apple sauce, not fresh apples.
3. Calcium is mopped up before lead in the digestive tract, so high levels will act as a buffer against lead absorption. But *don't* fall into the trap of taking lots of dairy products. Besides being mucus-forming, they actually *increase* lead absorption. Stick to other natural sources of calcium: bonemeal, alfalfa, sesame seeds, camomile, parsley, wheatgerm etc. (See page 95 on calcium.) Take 800 mg daily.
4. Vitamin E is known to be a protective agent in metal toxicity, but don't go above 800-1000 IUs and before you start adding it to your diet read the section on vitamin E again (pages 89-93). There are some contra-indications there which just may apply to you.
5. Vitamin C is an extremely powerful antitoxin – take a minimum of 3 g daily.
6. Vitamin A helps to activate the enzymes needed to detoxify poisonous metals, so eat plenty of the golden, orange and red plants and, if taking a supplement, combine A and D: 25,000-50,000 IUs daily of A with appropriate balancing amounts of D – 2,500-5,000 IUs. Take this for one week only at the beginning of each of the 3 months so that your liver doesn't get overburdened with it. It'll store what it doesn't immediately need.
7. A couple of cloves of raw garlic in a salad dressing or, if this is too anti-social, 6 garlic perles daily with meals. Like the seaweeds, these are also rich in the sulphur-containing amino acids. If you can't stand garlic use onions instead, but you'll need more, about two daily, best in onion soup. Or you could use half a cup of cooked legumes or beans daily

instead, which will carry out the same task. Finally, take 3 cups of detoxifying tea daily for six days a week.

Rest for one day then begin the cycle again and continue to do so for 3 months in all.

Detoxifying tea

     3 parts gipsy weed (*Lycopus europaeus*)
     3 parts yellow dock (*Rumex crispus*)
     ½ part plantain (*Plantago spp*)
     ½ part Jamaican ginger (*Zingiber officinale*)

Follow this programme for three months. And of course try and get aluminium out of your life and avoid lead by living away from the centre of a town or main road if possible. Certainly don't bring up your children within 200 yards of a motorway. Be careful where you buy your vegetables. It seems that those grown within a ten mile radius of Marble Arch are unfit for human consumption.

CHAPTER 4

Growing, Buying and Preparing Herbs

Some excellent books have been written about herb growing and those I like best I've listed in the appendix (page 296). I grow some 200 herbs in my own garden – this may sound formidable, but many of them are wildings which arrived uninvited but are nonetheless treasured. The ones I've conscientiously encouraged flourish in spite of me (for I'm sausage-fingered not green-thumbed as far as plants are concerned), so it's just as well that herbs are generally very tough. Once established they tend to romp away and look after themselves. They do have a few dislikes.

The woody herbs can survive constant wind, but most other herbs appreciate the protection of a wall, hedge or fence. Most like plenty of sunshine, though a few like parsley, chives, lovage, chervil, houseleek and most mints enjoy moist, partly sheltered sites. Herbs dislike being planted near voracious tree roots which rob them of valuable nutrients so they grow tall, thin and straggly.

Soil

Most herbs prefer light soil. A cover of garden peat spread 2½ cm (1 inch) thick keeps the soil friable and actually saves you weeding by keeping the soil underneath dark. Better still, you'll need to water the garden much less frequently once it has good peat cover, and the peat will stop the soil cracking up as a result of extreme temperatures and prevent it from becoming waterlogged. Dampen the peat a little before applying it in the spring.

Do not overfeed the soil with instant chemical liquid or dissolvable powder fertilisers. Few herbs need much feeding and any nutrient they need should be organic. Remember, you're not growing herbs, like leeks, for their size so you can win prizes. The herbs richest in essential oils, minerals and vitamins are often the smallest and most unprepossessing.

Organic fertiliser

If you have an elderberry bush or a birch tree you'll find they are the ideal site for a compost heap, because the excretions from their roots, together with their fallen leaves, speed up fermentation, producing a light compost which is especially effective for revitalising the soil and which can also double as a replacement for peat. An efficient heap should measure 180 cm (6 ft) by 120 cm (4 ft) and should be enclosed by planks or wire netting fastened to stakes in the ground which is then lined with straw or old newspapers. These will rot into the heap in time and so will need renewing occasionally. The idea is to prevent currents of air keeping the edges cool. The heap should have its bottom firmly planted on the bare earth in order to admit the necessary soil bacteria which decomposes the waste. You'll need to get at it too, so one side of the compost heap should have moveable supports.

Small gardens can generally only accommodate one of those bins specially designed for rotting waste into compost. Compost can be made from just about anything – weeds, leaves, lawn clippings, newspapers, vacuum cleaner dust, feathers, hay, straw, raw or cooked leftover food. Spread the cocktail 10 cm (4in) thick and sandwich with layers of soil garnished with herbal activators like nettles, which are particularly good for helping the nitrogen bacteria break up decaying vegetable matter and the carbons in paper; seaweed which is rich in trace minerals; comfrey with its high calcium and nitrogen content, and yarrow which accelerates decomposition. Camomile will stop excessive acidification, salerian flowers will stimulate phosphorus activity, tansy adds valuable potassium. In all instances use the leaves and/or flowers, not the roots which are difficult to break down, and use about a dessertspoon per layer.

When the heap is 120 cm (4 ft) high put a lid of soil on it. The final result should be dark and crumbly. If you haven't got the time to do all this use Biohumus or Maxicrop which are both good organic acids.

Horsetail fertiliser and fungal repellent

Horsetail is particularly good for preventing mint rust and mildew and for deterring black spot. It is excellent for herbs suspected of having a root disease and for strengthening newly planted seedlings. Make a decoction using 45 g (1½ oz) to 3 litres (5 pints) of water. Strain and use it to spray foliage until it drips.

Nettle foliage feeder

Nettles are not only an excellent foliage feed for plants, they are an effective spray against mildew, black fly, aphids and plant lice. Prepare as for horsetail, that is, adding 45 g (1½ oz) to 3 litres (5 pints) of water, but once cool add a dessertspoonful of liquid soap to help the spray stick to the foliage.

Yarrow fertiliser

Yarrow is full of copper and contains useful amounts of potash, phosphates, chlorides and lime. The latter is particularly important for herbs because it acts as a reagent, and without it herbs cannot use the other nutritives in fertilisers. If your garden produces beautiful azaleas, camellias and rhododendrons it will need more lime added to the soil to grow herbs successfully. Mix lime with equal quantities of magnesium carbonate and dig it into the soil. Then use yarrow as a fertiliser (made up in the same way as horsetail fertiliser) to encourage your new seedlings.

Garlic powder sprinkled among newly sown seeds stops birds eating them, as do powdered dried mugwort, rue and southernwood. If you sprinkle the seeds themselves with any of these dried herbs before planting and leave them for a few days to absorb their aromas, it will prevent them from being eaten underground by slugs.

These fertilisers, foliage feeders and fungus and insect repellents can be used for herbs grown indoors. They can be put in a fine mist spray bottle and the foliage should be sprayed once a week until it drips to ensure good healthy growth.

Indoors

Even if you live in a city it is still possible to grow some of your herbs in tubs indoors. Don't pick or use herbs growing outdoors in a city as they will almost certainly be heavily contaminated with lead. So hanging baskets and window boxes are out, except for purely decorative purposes.

Don't squash your herbs in tiny pots. Large ones contain more soil which keeps the moisture longer and contains more bacteria, so the herbs come closer to their natural growing conditions. Use a well-balanced compost like John Innes No 2 or one of the modern proprietary soilless composts. Garden soil will not do. It tends to encourage fungal growth and becomes waterlogged, and if it's taken from the environs of a big city it may well contain unacceptably high levels of lead.

Water the herbs from below, using the saucer in which the pot stands, and throw out any surplus water after two hours. Do not fall into the trap of overwatering which tends to catch so many indoor gardeners bent on killing with kindness. Keep the room well-aired and do not put your herbs in draughts. Mints, woodruff, sweet cicely, lady's mantle, balm, houseleek and chervil grow quite well without direct sunlight, but all the others need a sunny windowsill and rotating from time to time to allow the whole plant to enjoy an equal share of the light. Pinch off the tops to encourage bushy growth. When you cut the herbs for your own use take only a few select sprigs here and there so that the plant does not get bald patches and look unbalanced.

Propagation from nursery seedlings

If you're just beginning to grow herbs, the best plan is to find a good herb nursery and buy some potted seedlings from them. The following herb farms supply seeds and herb seedlings by carrier or to personal callers. Many of them also supply their own organically grown dried herbs.

Hollington Nurseries Ltd, Woolton Hill, Newbury, Berks. Telephone: (0635) 253908. Mr S. Hopkinson.

Lathbury Park Herbs Gardens, Newport Pagnell, Bucks. Telephone: (0908) 610316. Mrs Allan. Personal delivery to London area only, otherwise visitors to collect.

Herbs from the Hoo, 46 Church Street, Buckden, Cambs. Telephone: (0480) 810818. Mr & Mrs R. Peplow.

The Old Tavern, Compton Drusdon, Sonerton, Somerset. Telephone: (0458) 42347. Mr A. Lyman-Dixon. Personal callers only.

Stoke Lacy Herb Garden, Nr Bromyard, Herefordshire. Telephone: (0432 78) 232. Mrs M. Hooper.

Iden Croft Herbs, Frittenden Road, Staplehurst, Kent. Telephone: (0580) 891432. Mrs D. Titterington.

Wells & Winter Limited, Mereworth, Maidstone, Kent. Telephone: (0622) 812491. Mr J. Wells.

Oak Cottage Herb Farm, Nesscliffe, Nr Shrewsbury, Shropshire. Telephone: (074 381) 262. Mrs R. Thompson.

Valeswood Herb Farm, Little Ness, Shrewsbury, Shropshire. Telephone: (0939) 260376. Mrs B. Keen.

Suffolk Herbs, Sawyers Farm, Little Cornard, Sudbury, Suffolk. Telephone: (0787) 227247.

The Walled Garden, Thornham Herbs, Thornham Mague, Nr Eye, Suffolk. Telephone: (037 983) 510. Ms J. Davies. Fresh plants personal callers only, otherwise dried medicinal herbs by post.

Yorkshire Herbs, The Herbs Centre, Middleton Tyas, Richmond, N. Yorks. Telephone: (032 577) 686. Mr H. E. Bates.

The Herb Garden, Thunderbridge, Nr Huddersfield, S. Yorks. Telephone: (0484) 602 993. Personal callers only.

Down to Earth, Streetfield Farm, Cade Street, Heathfield, East Sussex TN21 9BS.

As soon as you receive your seedlings open them and water them well. Once the herbs have four distinct leaves they can be moved to an open bed, but make the transition gradual. Leave them in their bags or pots outdoors in a sheltered place for a few days to get acclimatised. Then soak the seedling in its plastic bag or pot in water and, having let the excess drain out carefully, invert the package, holding it in one hand and covering the top soil with the other, fingers spread lightly apart to allow the seedling to poke out between them. Squeeze the parcel repeatedly until the herb and its rootlets embedded in the soil come out in one piece, or if plastic bags prove stubborn cut and carefully peel away. Then, with the herb firmly encased in its native soil, transplant it outdoors so that the bottom of the stem is a good 2½ cm (1 in) below the surface. Water it in the evening with a rose attachment.

Propagation from seed

Seeds must be fresh. Angelica seed must be absolutely fresh or it won't germinate. Instructions on the back of the packet will tell you when to grow. If it is early in the year and very cold, help the soil along by pouring hot water over it before planting to speed up the germination process. Boiling water will kill off the valuable living organisms in the soil so use hot water only. Parsley can be helped by soaking the seeds overnight in luke warm water to soften the hard seed coats.

Mix fine seeds in a little sand before planting to help them retain moisture and deter slugs. Sow in moist ground and water with a rose attachment fitted to the can or hose. Thin them out when they are 5 cm (2 in) high.

Propagation by cutting

Woody herbs like sage, lavender, rosemary and thyme respond well to this method. Cut or pull a 15 cm (6 in) new sprout from a sturdy plant just below the leaf bud or stem joint so the twig has a heel. Put it in some water mixed with rooting compound and watch for the tiny rootlets to appear, then transplant outdoors gently. Strip off the lower leaves and water generously. Keep the foliage damp with a mist sprayer. Soft-stemmed plants like mint and balm usually take a week or two to produce roots and woody ones like lavender may take nearly two months. This can be done in the spring or early autumn equally successfully.

Alternatively, place the cuttings round the edge of a large terracotta pot filled with a mixture of one-third rooting compound, one-third sand and one-third peat moss. Pat the mixture down firmly. Once you can see strong leaf growth you will know they have rooted. Leave, to be sure, for a week or two then transplant to an open bed having stripped off the old leaves.

Propagation by layering

Many herbs which creep close to the ground can be propagated by layering in the spring. This is even surer and simpler than the cutting method. Just take one of the still attached branches of the parent herb and bend it gently towards the earth. You may need to anchor it with a U-shaped piece of wire. Then water generously to encourage root growth to spread down into the soil from the point where the plant touches it. After several weeks you will see a complete new plant forming and after six weeks you can sever it from its parent plant and transplant it. Catmint, horehound, hyssop, marjoram, all the mints, rosemary, sage and all the thymes respond well to this method.

Picking herbs

Most wild herbs are more potent than fresh ones for medicinal use, but if you're picking any herb it is important to note the following points:

1. Don't pick plants from verges or fields which have been sprayed with chemicals, traffic fumes or animal excreta, or industrial waste. Above all don't pick herbs in cities or large towns. This way you'll avoid unwittingly poisoning yourself.
2. Be selective when you pick and never strip an area of any one herb. A few herbs judiciously picked at intervals will ensure their survival and their availability next year, for even annuals, if allowed to come to seed, can replant themselves.
3. Remember that harvesting is a two-way exchange. If you treat the herb gently and pick it carefully it will offer you its best. Don't strip off too much bark from a single tree,

and certainly don't sabotage the tree by picking it all off in
a circle. Coax wax and gums off gently with a small sharp
knife. Hook high branches down with a curved walking
stick to avoid breaking them. Cut stems, don't break them.
Be quiet and dextrous to avoid crushing and bruising.

4.   Avoid yellowing, insect-ridden, weary-looking plants
and those growing tightly packed together fighting for soil
and air space.

5.   Pick herbs at exactly the right time as far as you can, both
as far as the season, the time of day and the weather
conditions are concerned. All herbs should be gathered in
the morning, when the dew has dried and the weather is
fine, after a brief period of fine sunny weather. Don't water
flowers the day before you pick them. If necessary compile
a picking calendar to help you observe the seasons. Buds
should be gathered in the spring, leaves at the beginning of
the summer, flowers generally in mid-summer the
moment they've unfolded, and roots, barks and berries in
the autumn or early winter. Some herbs like sweet cicely
and feverfew will crop twice if cut back vigorously after
the first harvesting.

Herb identification

If you don't know what you're picking, leave it alone. Books
which I find invaluable for plant identification are listed in the
appendix on page 296. They are beautifully illustrated and give
clear descriptions, and some are light and portable enough to
take with you on your plant hunting expeditions.

It is also vital to know which part of the plant you are seeking.
The Tibetans, for example, are extremely meticulous about this.
We tend to be sloppier. Where they would select the style and
stigmas of a herb, we might use the whole flower. Yet it is
essential to appreciate that the active principles of a plant are *not*
equally distributed throughout.

Of all the plant organs, leaves and roots are generally richest in
active substances. The leaf above all is where the synthesis takes
place, for it is here one finds the numerous alkaloids, heterosides
and aromatic essences. Sugars, glucose, vitamins and aromatic
oils tend to congregate in the roots while the stem is mainly a
transit organ. The reproductive organs and their separate parts

throughout their stages of development contain glycosides, aromatic oils and many other valuable medicinal substances. So when I mention a plant for medicinal use, I always mean the leaf unless I specifically cite another part, like the bark, berry or flower. All of the rules I've cited are general and it is therefore extremely important that you have some elementary knowledge of a plant's structure before attempting to gather it. It isn't simply a question of recognising the particular botanical species, but also of knowing which organs produce the active substance. Again you'll find books helpful in this respect listed in the appendix.

Protected species

Wild plants first came under the protection of the law in 1975 when twenty-one species of rare plants were included in the Conservation of Wild Creatures and Wild Plants Act. A list of these plants may be obtained from the Conservation Department, Royal Botanic Gardens, Kew, Surrey. Also remember it is a criminal offence to dig up *any* British wild plant without the consent of the owner of the land on which it grows, and that some herbs grow only in certain areas, so if you dig them up you may be destroying their habitat for ever.

Picking herbs

Leaves should be clean and insect-free. If they're not, spray them thoroughly with water or garlic or horsetail tea several days before they're due to be picked. They should be harvested young just before the flowers open when they are richest in medicinal powers. Nipping them off without stems will also help the plant to thicken up.

Flowers should be picked the moment they open, before they've been pollinated. This way their essential oils will remain in the petals instead of being lost in the air. If you can avoid it don't actually touch the petals. Cut the flower heads off directly over a drying tray, snipping off any thick stalks as you go, because they tend to prolong the drying time.

Seeds should be gathered pod and all, having been left to sun-ripen on the plant. Wind dispersal doesn't usually happen before the plant leaves begin to yellow and fall. Catch them just before this moment to be sure they're ripe.

Bark should be gathered early in the spring or autumn when it is thick and juicy with sap and medicinal properties are at their highest. Concentrate on the bark of the larger branches of sturdy, well-established trees and take only small pieces here and there. If you strip off great sheets you may kill the tree, and certainly don't try attacking saplings.

Roots are best gathered in the autumn when the top of the plant is dying down. Lift them out carefully without cutting or bruising, wash them well under cold running water to free them from soil, cut off any little hair rootlets and dry carefully with a cotton tea towel.

Berries should be picked when they're lusciously glossy, well before they have any chance to turn mushy. Wear gloves and long sleeves if you're harvesting sharp-thorned plants; you'll find a walking stick useful for holding back stems.

Collecting equipment

I use big, flat, woven baskets which allow me to separate and keep track of my herbs, and a pair of stainless steel scissors. Aluminium taints and stains herbs. When you cut be quick and precise. Don't collect herbs in plastic carrier bags, which will only heat them up and trap any traces of moisture, resulting in a bedraggled mildewed harvest.

Drying

Most of us are prone to illness in the darkest parts of the year so it is important to have a good supply of green dried herbs available. Fresh herbs are always preferable to dry ones, which inevitably lose some of their characteristic smell and taste due to the evaporation of their essential oils, no matter how meticulous the drying process has been. These oils increase the production of white corpuscles and, used externally, improve the circulation of the blood to the skin. Some encourage perspiration, help soothe inflammation and are highly effective bacteriocides and disinfectants. So drying should be quick and efficient in order to conserve as much of these precious oils as possible. The woodier herbs will survive all winter if they're appropriately sheltered, so you can continue to pick these fresh.

Poorly dried herbs leached of their colour are useless medicinally and you can come unstuck in this area by:

1. *heating* – if herbs are left heaped up after picking they'll burn from the middle like a pile of lawn clippings
2. *bruising* or crushing when handling
3. *spreading too thickly*
4. *drying too slowly* or at too low a temperature
5. *drying too quickly* at too harsh a temperature or in full sunlight or strong wind which will cause fading.

Don't leave your herbs heaped up outside even for half an hour. The only exception to this is comfrey. I know Jill Davies of Thornham Herbs dries hers most successfully by harvesting in the evening and leaving it spread out on the grass all night before taking it indoors. Comfrey is a particularly fleshy plant and so benefits from this exceptional treatment.

Dry all herbs indoors in warm, dark, airy rooms (**not** garages, for obvious reasons). The only exceptions are sphagnum moss, which needs outdoor sun and wind (artificial heat spoils it), and nettles, which enjoy drying outdoors in fine weather. If you're drying herbs in a big way then a well-constructed drying shed is a must. These need not be expensive. Barbara Keen of the Valeswood Herb Farm has the best drying shed I've ever seen, heated by a simple, slow combustion stove with pipes similar to those used for heating greenhouses and with shuttered windows. She's been running it economically for more than forty years and turning out exquisitely dried herbs. She keeps the temperature steady between 90° and 100°F and herbs dry in a matter of days. Those which give out a great deal of moisture quickly, such as parsley, and those which are easily bruised like comfrey, foxglove and belladonna, henbane and elderflowers, are placed in the hottest part of the shed for quick intensive drying. The shed is also well-ventilated because drying herbs give off a tremendous amount of moisture. Herbs are turned at least once daily and the flaccid herbs – mint, henbane, belladonna, horehound, woodsage and foxglove – are treated especially gently. The hardier herbs – walnut, chestnut, rosemary and thyme – can stand lots of stirring up. When the herbs shrink a little (usually within two days) they are moved **downwards** to make room for more of the same species above. This must not-be done in reverse because the fresh herbs will dampen the drying ones. Barbara's excellent book about how to construct a drying shed was written during the war but is still available (see appendix, page 296).

All the above applies to small-scale domestic drying. Cheesecloth stretched over wooden frames makes ideal drying racks and can be placed in a warm, airy attic or an airing cupboard. Sturdy picture frames are ideal for this purpose.

Woodier herbs can be dried in **small** bunches and hung from hooks in a warm, dark room free from steam and condensation. I dry many of mine very successfully over my Aga cooker on the days when we're eating raw foods only. Remember not to muddle up your seed heads. An easy way to catch them is to surround the upside-down head with a paper bag, closed firmly around the stem with string. The top of the bag nearest the stem should be perforated to encourage air circulation.

My assistant has tried drying herbs in a microwave oven but without much success, though I'm told it can be done. I don't recommend it, nor do I endorse oven drying. It's a finely tuned oven indeed that can keep the temperature at a steady 90°F, since leaving the oven door partly ajar, as one must in order to ensure ventilation, results in disparate temperature flows. I have resorted to oven drying when the weather has been abysmal, trying to restrict it to roots and barks which require prolonged drying and should emerge hard enough to break. If they're pliable, leathery or spongy they need more drying time.

Seeds are ready when they crack easily between the fingernails; leaves and stalks when they feel crisp and crackly. If they fall to powder when touched they're overdone. Petals are dry when they lose their silky texture and feel paper thin. Ideally they should emerge pretty close to their original colour. Berries are ready when they shrivel up like currants; hawthorn berries require especially careful drying – don't overdo it or they'll become impossibly hard and so uncrushable. Sphagnum moss, having been collected in clumps and spread out to dry outdoors, should be shaken out and picked clean at least once, and when completely dry is best stored in loosely woven linen bags.

Storing

Never store herbs in plastic bags and avoid paper bags which are too easily nibbled by vermin and insects or attacked by mildew. Cotton or linen sacks are acceptable but need to be hung up and not left resting on a stone floor. The herbs in them should be inspected every week, examined for moth and stirred up from the bottom to test for dampness. If found wanting they should be redried, and make sure the container is also thoroughly dried.

I've always found the best storage equipment is glass jars with tightly fitted lids. They **must** be kept away from light and heat which will extract the active principles of the herbs and fritter them away in the surrounding air. So keep clean glass in a dark room (my medicinal herbs are stored in a darkened spare room in enormous, old-fashioned sweet jars). Failing that, you can always protect your herbs from light by using amber or green glass, but this tends to be more expensive. Glass is particularly good because you can see at a glance how fast you're using up the herb. Check herbs in glass periodically for dampness. Mildew spreads like wildfire. If you're storing herbs in quantity, well-made wooden boxes are ideal.

Label your herbs clearly, recording the month and the year when they were harvested, both the common and the Latin names of the plant and the part of the herb. Replace your stocks of dried herbs yearly and treat your compost heap to the residue. Barks and roots can be kept for two years.

Buying herbs

If it is impossible for you to grow your own herbs you can buy them in person or by mail order at the following suppliers:

Neal's Yard Apothecary, 2 Neal's Yard, Covent Garden, London WC2. Telephone: (01) 379 7662.

Baldwins, 173 Walworth Road, London SE17. Telephone: (01) 703 5550.

L'Herbier De Provence, 341 Fulham Road, London SW10. Telephone: (01) 352 0012.

Gerard House, 736 Christchurch Road, Boscombe, Bournemouth, Hants. Telephone: (0202) 35352.

Culpeper Ltd, Hadstock Road, Linton, Cambridge CB1 6NJ. Telephone: (0223) 891196. Branches in Brighton, Bath, Guildford, Norwich, Oxford, Salisbury and Winchester. Three branches in London.

D. Napier & Sons, 17/18 Bristol Place, Edinburgh, Scotland. Telephone: (031) 225 5542.

Down to Earth, 3 The Grove, Coulsdon, Surrey CK3 2BH.

Medicinal & Culinary Herbs, 26 Frodsham Street, Chester, Cheshire.

Many health food shops sell dried herbs but please check their quality to ensure they are carefully green-dried. Most of the farms that supply seeds and herb seedlings (see page 112) also supply very nicely dried herbs that they grow themselves. All these suppliers will answer queries on the phone but it is probably better to write for their catalogues enclosing a large stamped, addressed envelope.

Buying prepared herbal tablets is acceptable at a pinch, but by far the best approach is to make up your own formulations according to your own needs. The ones I offer in this book are those I've found particularly successful in my own practice, but they are not written on tablets of stone. It is perfectly acceptable to substitute alternative herbs, but don't do this unless you're very sure of their comparative properties. If in any doubt at all seek the advice of a qualified medical herbalist. If you're buying herbal pills, check that they don't contain synthetic chemical preservatives like potassium sorbate or sulphur dioxide, artificial colours, starch, sugar, lactose, cellulose, silicon dioxide, stearates or gluten. If the assistant in the shop doesn't know, write and ask the manufacturer. Don't assume they don't contain them just because the label only lists the active ingredients. Many of the additives in herbal tablets are capable of upsetting the digestive tract and you should take your herbs as uncontaminated as possible.

Some shops will sell you a herbal fluid extract or tincture over the counter if you're prepared to have a stand up, quick consultation, but please be careful. If the problem is even slightly worrying, it is far preferable to have a proper professional consultation otherwise you may finish up treating the symptoms and not getting to the root of the problem and treating the cause.

No responsible qualified medical herbalist will treat you by post. You'll need to have at least two or three consultations to ensure an accurate diagnosis and some follow-up. Check on the cost of the consultation and its duration before you go, as prices vary widely.

It may certainly be possible to show a formulation to an assistant in a health food shop and have it made up for you. Much depends on the policy of the shop. Practising medical herbalists will insist on making up a formulation of their own for you, so please don't wave this book at such a person and ask for a specific formula. Your formulation will be carefully tailored to cope with your condition.

Equipment for preparation

Nothing makes me more irritated than people who think a sprinkle of herbs in hot water is going to do them good. For herbs to be effective they **must** be taken in the right dose, so accurate kitchen scales which will measure small quantities of ½oz upwards are essential. Those with a large weighing pan are needed to weigh out bulky fresh herbs. Some home-brewing shops sell mini-balances which are useful, as are the old-fashioned portal weighing scales for measuring powdered herbs. Herbs should never be contaminated with metal, particularly copper, lead or aluminium. Use stainless steel knives and scissors, glass, enamel, pottery, bone and stainless steel containers, saucepans, sieves and spoons. Bottles should be glass, preferably amber or green (certainly never plastic), with ground glass or cork stoppers. Essential oils are so powerful they'll eat into plastic.

You'll need an eye dropper for measuring out these oils and a flexible palette knife. If you're using pottery or porcelain saucepans you'll need a heat diffusing mat to protect them from cracking.

Choose a good solid pestle and mortar. Herbs need weight behind them to be effectively crushed. A flimsy mortar will bounce all over the kitchen table. Glass ones scratch easily so avoid them. I use a Japanese suribachi made of stoneware with the grooves running in wedge shapes set at differing angles inside the mortar, and I clean it with a birch twig brush. It is efficient but suribachi are difficult to get hold of. You may be lucky enough to find them in the more enlightened wholefood shops. Failing that, use the pestle and mortar generally used by chemists and the pottery industry. They're widely available and comparatively inexpensive, and pestles and mortars never wear out.

Use big muslin squares dropped inside sieves for filtering, or coffee filter paper for small quantities. Muslin should always be sterilised by boiling after use, dried and then carefully stored in a paper bag for protection. A coffee grinder is helpful for grinding up tough dried berries. Don't forget your self-adhesive labels.

Quantities

It is essential to measure out herbs according to prescription, but bear in mind the following points:

1. All doses in this book are for adults of average body weight of between 10 and 11 stone. Women weighing less than this should decrease the dose proportionately.

2. It is important to dose a child accurately and a useful rule to ensure this is to divide a child's **next** birthday by 24. So the dose for a seven-year-old would be $8/24 = 1/3$ of adult dose.

3. Babies generally prefer herbs applied externally; these are then absorbed internally through the skin. This can be done by massaging creams or oils into the skin, by immersing the baby in a herbal bath (**not** including the face of course!) or by osmosis through the hands and feet in small foot/hand baths. Alternatively, herbs can be administered using an enema, but in my experience most children and babies don't take fondly to this unless they're so sick they haven't the strength to protest.

Always bear in mind that most herbs lose about eighty per cent of their weight while drying, so 5 lbs of fresh are needed to produce 1 lb of dried; with the woody stemmed herbs the proportion is about 4:1. Parsley takes 10 lbs of fresh to produce 1 lb of dried, and flowers and the very watery plants are 20:1. All quantities in this book are for dried, not fresh, herbs.

Water

When water is called for in any medicinal preparation use pure bottled spring or filtered water (see below), not water straight from the tap which is laden with chemicals.

Medicinal herbal teas

These are the simplest way to take herbs and, if taken faithfully in the right quantities, are extremely effective. If using dried herbs avoid finely powdered ones which are hard to filter and produce a muddy unappetising soup. Use dried herbs which have been chopped or crumbled instead. Fresh herbs should be gently crushed to break up the cellulose of the plant cells, so releasing the active principles. You can do this with a knife, in your hands, or with a pestle and mortar.

Keep a special teapot aside for medicinal teas. Ordinary teapots get stained with tannin and should you be brewing, for example, a tea of iron-rich herbs, the iron from these and the tannic acid from the staining will bond together to form tannate of iron, a very powerful styptic which causes acute constipation and tummy problems. The quantities for a medicinal herbal tea are always the same, one ounce to one pint of boiling filtered water. From this you'll be able to draw about 1½ cups of tea, which is generally taken ½ cup at a time with meals during the day. Remember one ounce of fresh herb will look considerably more than the same quantity of dried herb, so don't be alarmed by the visual difference – it's the accurate weight that's important.

Infusions

Delicate parts of a herb, like the flowers and leaves, need to be gently steeped in water for twenty minutes. Begin by warming the pot you save for herbal tea making; add one ounce of the dried herb or proportionately more of the crushed fresh herb and pour over one pint of water that has been brought to a rolling boil. Cover the pot tightly to stop the valuable volatile oils escaping in the evaporating steam. Leave to steep and strain (through muslin, nylon, silver or stainless steel strainer) and drink. Store the residue in the refrigerator in a glass container covered with linen or muslin. It can be kept like this for three days. After this it may start fermenting and should be thrown away on your compost heap. You can tell when it does – fine bubbles start to pop up to the surface and the tea begins to smell brackish.

Sun-steeped tea can be made in the same way in a glass container, using cold water. Put the container in a very hot, sunny spot and leave it to steep for two to three hours, remembering to keep it tightly covered. A herbal tea drunk purely for pleasure will only need to be steeped for a few minutes, depending on how strong you want the flavour to be.

Decoction

This is made from seeds, roots, barks or very leathery leaves (like bay leaves) which, because of their toughness, need more rigorous processing to give up their properties. A decoction therefore has to be boiled. Herbs rich in volatile oil should be simmered in a tightly covered saucepan. Most other herbs need to be simmered in a partly covered saucepan for twenty minutes until the one pint of water originally added is reduced to approximately half that quantity. Strain and drink, and expect the resulting brew to taste pretty strong. I prefer an enamel-lined saucepan for decoctions, but any other type will do providing it isn't aluminium or lined with Teflon.

Seeds, roots and barks will need vigorous crushing in a pestle and mortar before brewing. Burdock root and cinnamon only need steeping in freshly boiled water, not boiling, and valerian root should be steeped in *cold* water for twenty-four hours to ensure the valerianic acid and essential oils in the root are not dissipated. Decoctions stay fresh longer than infusions, generally for up to four days, and should be stored in the fridge.

To make a double-strength infusion or decoction simply

double the amount of herb used and keep the same quantity of water as for a single-strength mixture. To make a quadruple-strength infusion or decoction increase the original amount of herb used four times and use the same quantity of water.

Macerations

Water, oil, cider vinegar, white wine vinegar, wine, vodka, brandy and gin are all suitable liquids in which to macerate herbs. The results, depending on which you use, are all given different names.

Cold water maceration is not often used as, not surprisingly, it tends to be a rich breeding ground for bacteria. If using this don't leave the herbs for more than twelve hours before straining and refrigerating. Grain macerations for digestive purposes need longer (see page 17).

Essential oils are not difficult to make. Pound to a pulp two ounces of freshly picked herb (the dried will have lost much of its innate essential oil already so is less useful) with a pestle. Scrape it into a wide-necked glass container and cover with one pint of vegetable oil, the best being sweet almond, sesame or, failing that, olive oil. Add a tablespoon of cider vinegar to help the continuing breaking up of the cellulose of the herb and make sure the jar is still only three-quarters full so there is room to shake the mixture vigorously. Do this and place outside in strong sunlight embedded in fine sand which will attract and hold sun heat for hours after the sun has gone down. Bring the jar in at night and shake again vigorously, storing it in the airing cupboard. In the winter use the airing cupboard throughout the process. Keep this up for a week then strain and bottle the oil. If it is not strong enough (and you can judge this by its fragrance when rubbed on a pulse point) repeat the process all over again using the same oil and cider vinegar but a fresh batch of herbs.

The process can be speeded up by using artificial heat but I don't think the results are quite as good. Place the closed jar in a pan of freshly boiled water and try to keep it just below the boil for two hours. This is more difficult than it sounds, and you'll need to top up the water from time to time. Strain and bottle when cool. Some herbalists add a drop or two of vitamin E oil as an antioxidant to ensure preservation, but if the original oil was of superior quality this is generally unnecessary.

Wine maceration – Follow the same procedure as for essential oil but use one ounce of herb to one pint wine and macerate in sunlight for three days only. Artificial heat is not advisable. Use wine or better still cider vinegar, which is rich in trace minerals, particularly potassium. Such vinegars are also helpful used externally for itchy skin and some skin disorders, as they help to balance the pH of the skin, so restoring its protective acid mantle. Store in dark glass bottles and stopper firmly. Vinegar macerations are ideal for herbs which contain valuable gums and balsamic resins which will not dissolve in water.

Alcoholic macerations or tinctures can be made with brandy, gin or vodka. The alcohol used must be of good quality. Cheap alcohol will hurt the liver. Under no circumstances should cheap surgical spirit be used. The final concentration of alcohol in the tincture should be one-third, and alcohol is useful because it will normally extract all the important ingredients from a herb whereas water often won't. They will also keep indefinitely, and are useful for some of the terrible-tasting herbs or those that need to be taken over a prolonged period. Combine four ounces of powdered or very finely chopped herbs with one pint of alcohol. Shake daily, allowing the herb to extract for two weeks exactly.

Tinctures should be started with a new moon and strained with a full moon fourteen days later so that the power of the waxing moon will help extract the herbal properties to the utmost degree. I've found tinctures made outside of this syncopation significantly less effective. Strain the herb, particularly if it's powdered, through a finely woven muslin cloth. Bottle and cap tightly. The amount of alcohol ingested with a tincture is very small, but for those who cannot cope with it use the vinegar maceration instead. Tinctures are generally taken 5 ml (ie a level teaspoon) three times daily with meals.

Juices

Use fresh clean herbs only for this and extract the juice in a juicer. Add only a teaspoon at a time to a large glass of strongly flavoured vegetable or fruit juice (pineapple or tomato for example) as the taste is very pungent. Such juices can also be used externally as a compress or part of a dressing. They'll keep stored in the refrigerator in glass overnight, but not longer, and storing is inadvisable as much of the water-soluble vitamins will have evaporated.

Powders

Use perfectly dry herbs and put them through a coffee grinder, then sieve or use a food processor with a very powerful motor to chop them finely. Herbs can sometimes be bought powdered, and spices are generally already powdered, but these will have lost much of the lingering remains of essential oil. Powders can be mixed with honey to a thick paste, rolled on a marble slab into thin sausages, cut into pellets and rolled into balls, then lightly sprinkled with slippery elm to avoid the pills sticking together and facilitate their digestion. Those suffering from hypoglycaemia (and I believe it is one of the twentieth century's epidemic diseases which goes largely unrecognised), those with pancreatic problems like diabetes, and people trying to lose weight should *not* take powdered herbs in this way. Use gelatin capsules instead.

Gelatin capsules

These vary in size, but generally adults use the '00' size and children the '0' size. The two parts of the capsule are separated and the open ends are pressed into the powdered mixture repeatedly and firmly until the open halves of the capsule are as full as possible. Press the powder well in with a fingertip and carefully close the capsule by pressing the two ends together so one side slots into the other. This method of ingestion is ideal for the more powerful herbs which need to be taken in small quantities of a half to four grams at a time. Capsules are *always* taken with meals and washed down with purified water or herbal tea. If more than one prescription is to be taken, leave a fifteen minute gap between dosages. Occasionally prescriptions like herbal antibiotics need to be taken on an empty stomach, in which case use generous amounts of herbal tea or water to facilitate their digestion.

Some of my patients prefer to measure out their powder with the capsule into some yoghurt or sugarless jam (like the 'Whole Earth' varieties), but be prepared for some strong tastes! Personally, I prefer this method as it ensures the herb is properly digested, beginning with the ptyalin in the saliva, but many patients cannot stomach the strong taste.

Pills

Pills are useful when the herb cannot be finely powdered but can be coarsely chopped and is strong and needs to be taken in small quantities. Mix the coarsely powdered herbs with an added tenth of marshmallow or slippery elm and carefully dribble in cold purified water, stirring hard all the time until a dough is formed. Roll out on a marble slab into thin sausages, then cut into pellets and shape into pea-size balls. Spread on a stainless steel baking sheet and dry out overnight in an airing cupboard. Such pills are equivalent to half the dose of a size '0' capsule, so adults will generally need to take four in place of their single '00' capsule.

Syrups

Syrups should always be made with honey not sugar because sugar gives nothing but empty calories, besides which it has an irritating habit of turning to caramel as soon as you take your eyes off it. Honey is better for you as the bees have thoughtfully pre-digested it, so it is easily assimilated. It is naturally antiseptic and antibiotic, and it doesn't cause the blood sugar to rocket in a reasonably healthy person (that is one without hypoglycaemia or diabetes) to higher levels than can easily be coped with by the body. Rapid absorption by the human body prevents fermentation. Finally, it is generally rich in vitamin C (depending on the type of nectar from which it came) and some B vitamins, and is groaning with trace minerals and some enzymes. Use dark local honey if you can get it, as it will be richer in vitamins and minerals than imported honey.

Remember that honey contains the properties of those flowers on which the bees have fed. So the famous thyme honey disinfects the throat and lungs, heather honey helps the urinary system, lime blossom honey is soothing, rosemary honey stimulating, and clover and orange blossom honeys are particularly good for coughs and sore throats. As a syrup is generally used for soothing coughs and sore throats, use these last two if you can.

To make a herbal syrup first prepare a double-strength decoction (see page 126), cool, strain and weigh it. Then pour it into an enamel saucepan and stir in a quarter its weight in honey. Thicken slowly over a low heat, stirring gently until the mixture turns syrupy. Skim off any rising scum from time to time. Bottle in glass and take a teaspoon as needed. Children will only need about half a teaspoon and will appreciate flavouring from licorice, anise seed or wild cherry bark as part of the formula.

Electuaries for children

This is a useful way of disguising unpalatable herbs in pounded dried fruits and honey or maple syrup, sugarless jams, carob chocolate and nut pastes. Administering these is a delicate balance between enticing presentation and imaginative disguise, of which more in the chapter on children's ailments.

Poultices

These are a very useful way of applying herbs externally. First clean the skin thoroughly with an antiseptic herbal decoction. Spread a large piece of cotton gauze onto a large china plate and place this on top of a saucepan of simmering water so that the underside is heated. Have a quadruple-strength unstrained decoction or infusion of your choice simmering alongside, and slowly add enough coarse slippery elm powder with one hand while stirring hard with the other to form a paste. Spread the warm paste on half the gauze, keeping it from the edge otherwise it will squelch out when you use it. Fold the other half of gauze over the top and pinch, then fold the damp edges together. Lay the gauze over the affected part of the body, making sure it is bearably hot and will not scald the skin – 45°C (113°F) is the ideal temperature. Cover it with a sheet of plastic to trap in the moisture as long as possible.

Change the poultice every five minutes, putting the old one

back on the plate to warm up again so you're re-using one of two poultices for the duration of the treatment. A series of short applications with breaks in between is much more effective than one long, uninterrupted application. It is invaluable for drawing out poison from the skin, relieving inflammation and promoting proper blood flow and so cleansing the area. Linseed, comfrey, plantain and marshmallow may all be used for this purpose and their action can be promoted by adding a small proportion of a herbal stimulant like ginger, mustard or cayenne. It is also possible to moisten the herbs with apple cider vinegar, plain hot water or one of the flower waters. If a continual flow of pus needs to be encouraged, use drawing herbs like slippery elm and linseed.

Mini-poultices are easily applied outdoors for emergencies like bites and stings. Pick clean leaves of plaintain, marshmallow, vine or geranium and chew rapidly to a pulp, mixing with plenty of saliva and not swallowing. Spread over the swelling and, if you have a strip of plastic or cotton, cover it with this to hold it in place until the patient can be helped indoors.

Fomentations or compresses

These are liquid versions of a poultice used externally to encourage the circulation of lymph or blood to a specific area, so relieving swellings, aches and colds. Make sure the skin is scrupulously clean and swab it down with antiseptic herbal tea such as thyme or sage. Dip a cotton towel or flannel in a warm (not scalding) infusion or decoction, wring it out lightly and spread over the affected area. Cover with plastic and a hot water bottle or an electric heating pad (making sure there is no danger of it shorting, which there won't be as long as the pad is perfectly dry and there is moisture between the body and the dry heat). Sip an appropriate herbal tea to help the healing process.

Alternate hot and cool poultices revitalise the body and are particularly good for sprained muscles. Leave the cool poultice on for five minutes only at a time. Fomentations can also be made from warmed oils, expressed plant juices, tinctures and fluid extracts.

Dressings

These are simply thin herbal **pastes** made from minced herbs spread on gauze and applied directly to the skin. Use only mild herbs for this. Powerful herbs applied directly to the skin may burn or irritate and need the brake of an added layer of cloth (as in a poultice). These should be renewed every two hours for the first day. After that they can be left longer but never for more than twelve hours. If using a comfrey bandage you'll notice bits may adhere to the skin. If this happens, leave it on and spread fresh comfrey paste on top as comfrey contains a cell proliferant which will help to form new skin.

Vaginal douches

When I mention douching to many of my patients they look apprehensive, but douches, used sensibly and in moderation, are an excellent way to keep the vagina healthy. They cut down the incidence of vaginitis, which two out of every three suffer from at some time during their lives, and relieve painful periods. Like enemas, they are very active, so use only mild herbs for these, well strained, at body temperature – 37°C (78°F). Never take more than two douches daily, and this only in cases of stubborn infection and stop them as soon as it clears up, otherwise the delicate balance of natural bacteria in the vagina will be disturbed. Maintain the pH balance by adding a tablespoon of cider vinegar or a teaspoon of fresh lemon juice to each quart of infusion or decoction. In my experience plain yoghurt, although much recommended by other manuals, seems to cause even worse irritation with my patients. Perhaps they've just been unlucky, but go carefully with yoghurt. Begin by making sure your douche kit is scrupulously clean. Vaginal douche kits can be bought from more enlightened chemists and from myself (see appendix page 296). Make an infusion or decoction, depending on the herb used, strain and allow to cool to the right temperature. Hang the bag which has a strong hook attachment on the wall next to the bath two feet (not more) above the hips. Insert the nozzle 1½ in into the vagina, release the clamp slowly so it doesn't rush in, and let it run in and drain out. Retain for ten to twenty minutes (see page 278). Needless to say pregnant women should *never* douche.

Enemas

These are used to treat nervousness, pain, fevers, to cleanse the bowel, relieve inflammation and as a means of carrying nourishment into the body. For those who are not just nervous but horrified at the thought of such invasive treatment, let me reassure you. Firstly, such a treatment is quite logical. You wouldn't try to unblock a kitchen drain from the top of the waste pipe, would you? Nor should a blocked colon be relieved from the top end by mouth only. It is also imperative to relieve the bowel of as much toxic waste as possible quickly by means of an enema in the event of a fever. If you're so weak you can't eat, then a certain amount of nourishment can be taken from an enema of spirulena or slippery elm. Secondly, enemas really are comfortable and easy to administer. I've had patients get themselves into a dreadful tangle through sheer nervousness, but if you lay everything out in advance and give yourself plenty of time, you'll find administering an enema is easy and the more relaxed you are the easier it is. Thirdly, enemas do not make a mess. Your anal sphincter muscle will hold the liquid in the colon until you're ready to release it. Initially the stimulus the enema fluid gives the bowel may make you want to rush straight to the toilet and release it, but you'll get better and gain more self-control with practice.

Adults will eventually find they can accept up to two litres of fluid into the colon, children less according to age. Use cool enemas to clean out the bowel and warm ones for treating nervousness. Fill up the bag with a strained tea, then lie on your right side in the bath or on a rug protected with a sheet of plastic and gently press the lubricated tip of the enema tube into the rectum. Release the clamp and allow the liquid to flow slowly into the rectum. If it encounters a block of impacted faeces turn off the tap, massage the area, go up into a shoulder stand to encourage the flow and then lie down again and inject more tea. Initially you may have a great urge to void, but this is only because the bowel's elasticity is so poor, and with practice you'll get better. Try to retain for twenty minutes and release. Enemas should *always* be taken while fasting, but should not be overused or relied on in place of a proper bowel movement.

Pessaries

This is really just a shaped internal poultice made by adding enough finely powdered herbs to gently warmed cocoa butter to

form a dough, which is then shaped in sausage shapes ¾ in thick
and 1½ in long and rounded at the end for easy insertion.
Alternatively, slippery elm moistened with water can be used as
a carrier base. The pessaries can be individually wrapped in
waxed paper and should be refrigerated or kept very cool. Once
unwrapped, they should be inserted as high into the rectum or
vagina as possible before bed. Body heat will then gently release
the herbs. Protect the sheets with a towel and wear cotton
knickers and, if necessary, a sanitary towel, and rinse the anus or
vagina well the next morning.

Pessaries are useful for astringing, soothing, cleansing,
drawing out poisons and carrying herbs to the requisite area
internally to treat infections, irritations, cysts, tumours and
haemorrhoids.

Baths

Herbs can be ingested into the body through the skin by osmosis,
and herbal baths, to be effective, need to be strong. They are
particularly good for soothing or stimulating the circulation
depending on the type of herbs used, and as a way of getting
herbs into the system if the body is very weak. Hand and foot
baths are easier to prepare and work even more effectively,
because the extremities are the most receptive parts of the body.

Add a strong, unstrained decoction of herbs to equal
quantities of freshly boiled water, pouring it into an enamel or
china or glass container. Immerse feet into the bath for eight
minutes first thing in the morning before eating. Hand baths
should be taken before supper for the same length of time. In both
instances the baths should be bearably hot but not boiling.

For baths add a gallon of strained decoction to a medium filled
bath and immerse as much as possible of the body under water
for twenty minutes, supporting the head on a bath pillow. Don't
use soap. Make sure the skin is clean *before* climbing into the
bath by vigorously skin brushing (see page 150) using a dry brush
on a dry skin. Really dirty bits can be washed with an organic
soap.

Gargles

These should be used as hot as possible to be effective and can be made from infusions, decoctions, macerations, tinctures and diluted, salted, pressed juices to relieve sore mouths and throats.

Eye baths

Should be made from very gentle herbs like cornflowers, marigolds, eyebright or raspberry in weak infusions. They should always be freshly made, meticulously strained, and applied lukewarm using a sterilised eye bath and changing the wash for each eye. Treat both eyes, even if only one is troubling you. Alternatively, particularly for children, apply warm compresses and change frequently.

Ointments

Used for their protective emollient effects and usually made by combining melted beeswax or cocoa butter with herbal oils which can be bought and which, when cooled, form a thick, spreadable paste. Wheatgerm or simple tincture of benzoin or myrrh may be added (5 drops to 250 ml) to help preserve it, though if the ointment is kept covered with waxed paper this is not usually necessary. Use 1 pint of herbal oil to about 2 oz of melted beeswax. When applying ointments externally be generous and rub them in thoroughly. Beeswax gives a stiff, slimy consistency, cocoa butter a richer oily one.

Liniments

These are thinner than ointments (and are usually made with a touch of oil dissolved in alcohol or vinegar). They are used for their rubefacient effect as a counter-irritant on the skin to penetrate the muscles, warming and relaxing them. They are especially helpful as part of the treatment for arthritis and for certain types of inflammation. When massaged into the skin, the alcohol will quickly evaporate, but the herbs will have penetrated the skin.

Creams

Creams are lighter versions of ointments which are excellent for treating sore or chapped skin. Children and babies usually prefer them as they are easier to apply. 1 oz of beeswax or cocoa butter to 4 fl oz of herbal oil and 1 fl oz of flower water (elderflower, witchhazel, orange flower, rosewater). First melt the beeswax in a double boiler, beat in the oil with a wooden spoon and, having removed the pan from the heat, slowly trickle in the flower water, beating hard until the cream cools. Vegetable glycerine, which is an excellent humescent, may be substituted for flower water. Both ointments and creams should be stored in wide-necked jars, and creams should be kept in the fridge to prolong shelf life. You can use the same preservative as in ointments, adding them in with the flower water.

Burning herbs

Herbs can be burned to purify the air – in Malaya cinnamon sticks are burned in birthing huts to relieve the pain of labour. Herbs can be smoked in a pipe or a water pipe to relieve bronchial congestion and coughs and, unlike tobacco, do not contain addictive nicotine. Some herbs can be smoked to treat insomnia and nervousness, but even herbs can produce irritating particles and tar as they burn. I prefer to administer soothing teas, massages and baths for this problem. When smoking, draw the inhaled fumes as deeply into the lungs as possible, then breathe out fully and completely. Do this only eight times in all at any one session.

Storing your formulations

Anything made with alcohol or vinegar will keep for well over a year if stored in firmly stoppered opaque glass bottles, but do remember that any herbal mixture, no matter how effectively dried or preserved, will grow less effective with age. So throw out any dried herbs once they've passed their first birthday. Syrups will keep indefinitely as honey is such an excellent preservative, but should be stored in the fridge tightly covered, preferably with a vacuum seal. Essential oils will keep indefinitely in small, sterilised opaque glass bottles but air gaps should be eliminated by transferring them to smaller and smaller jars as they get used up. Poultices and compresses should always be freshly made, and cotton or gauze bandages should be well boiled after use, dried and stored in sealed plastic bags. If they've become sticky with ointment throw them out.

Herbal preparations which have 'gone off' begin to smell odd, fizz or turn ominous colours, in which case your compost heap will still be grateful for their libation. Always sterilise containers before use with a thorough boiling, and screw on sterilised lids or plug uncapped bottles with generous wads of cotton wool. Corks should first be softened in boiling hot water and then sterilised in diluted vinegar.

If all these instructions seem too complicated, please don't be put off. It really is reasonably easy and the results are certainly worth the trouble, in terms of efficacy. Begin with the simplest ways of taking herbs, in infusions, decoctions and baths, and when you feel confident you've mastered the art of making these correctly, move on to the more adventurous ointments, pessaries and essential oils. Many herbal suppliers will send these already made up, but there's a special joy in having your own comfrey ointment in the family medicine chest awaiting emergencies, for example. It's like the difference between shop bought and home-made cake, besides which you can guarantee its quality, knowing you've put the best possible ingredients in at the highest practical percentages.

CHAPTER 5

Cleansing the Body

How to begin a herbal treatment

The first step is to open up the five eliminative channels of the body and flush out all the poisons that have been stopping its proper functioning. The only exception to this beginning is if you are very weak, elderly, or run down because you've had the illness for a long time. In this instance you'll need to first build up the body through improved nutrition and use large quantities of herbs which are mild in action, only embarking on an eliminative programme once you are strong enough to cope with it. In all instances, herbs should be included in copious quantities in the diet, which is why I've spent so much time on herbs as nutrition. If you're too ill to eat, then take them in juices, oil massage, baths, vaporised oils and steam compresses, pessaries or enemas. (Chapter 4 gives instructions on the preparation of all these.) If you are elderly, or particularly fragile, or have suffered from an illness for a long time you're best advised to seek the help of a medical herbalist. If in doubt with babies, administer herbs externally only in hand and foot baths, full baths or by massage using diluted essential oils.

Length of treatment

Be patient and persistent. When I talk to some of my chronically ill patients, I feel sorely in need of a ten-foot flashing neon sign saying 'Rome wasn't built in a day'. An illness that's taken years to insinuate itself into the body will take a long time to root out, and the person concerned will also need gradually to adjust a lifetime of habits and attitudes that induced the illness in the first place. In other words, getting well the natural way is hard work if you've been ill for some time. It's also challenging and it can be fun. The general rule of thumb is to allow a month of treatment for every year the disease has been working its way into your life, and remember – the time when the symptoms appeared is just the tip of the iceberg. If the illness is acute, like a bad cold, a gastric upset or a burn, it is generally self-correcting and will pass fairly quickly. By all means help it with herbs; don't suppress it with chemical drugs, and make some rapid adjustments to the diet (usually by fasting). Don't make the mistake of stopping the treatment abruptly as soon as you're back to normal again. Continue it for at least a fortnight to ensure its good effects are thoroughly assimilated by the body. In this way you'll be shielding yourself from a repeat attack.

Measurements

When one part is stated in a herbal formulation always assume this to be 1 oz or 28 g. So when you measure out your herbs, weigh them accurately. If one herb is bulkier than the rest and it seems you are weighing them accurately and adding a handful of this to a teaspoon of something else, don't be dismayed and shy off thinking you've got it wrong. That's the way it should be and you *are* making up the herbal formulation correctly.

Fresh versus dried herbs

Both are equally acceptable, though fresh herbs are better for reasons outlined on page 118. However, there's no doubt about it, dried herbs are far more convenient. Don't be phased by quantity. Fresh herbs are always much bulkier than dried ones.

Which parts of the herb to use?

Always use the dried or fresh leaf unless specifically asked to do otherwise. This applies throughout this book.

The body's channels

The five great eliminative channels of the body are the bowel, the skin, the lungs, the kidneys and the lymphatic system. But there are also smaller orifices which are used – the ears, eyes, the navel, the vagina in women, and on a slower basis, nails and hair.

The bowel

I'm often teased by friends for being totally obsessed with bowel movements, but the bowel is one of our biggest eliminative organs and should dump pounds of waste every day, and constipation is one of the major bug-bears of the Western world. A lot of people think that if they have a bowel movement once or even three times a day they are not constipated, but most of these people are failing to eliminate four-fifths of the food they ingest every ten hours. Dr Jensen cites a startling statistic: 'While attending the National College in Chicago many years ago, autopsies were performed on 300 persons. According to the history of these persons, 285 had claimed they were not constipated and had normal movements, and only fifteen had admitted they were constipated. The autopsies showed the opposite to be the case however, and only fifteen were found not to have been constipated, while 285 were found to have been constipated. Some of the histories of these 285 persons stated they had had as many as five or six bowel movements daily, yet autopsies revealed that in some of them the bowels were 12 inches in diameter. The bowel walls were encrusted with material (in one case peanuts) which had been lodged there for a long time', *Intestinal Disorders, Fasting and Eliminative Diets*, publishing division of Bernard Jensens Products, Solana Beach, California, 1980, p6.

A healthy bowel needs plenty of pure water without any chemicals or additives. It needs good nerve and muscle tone, adequate circulation, and excellent nutrition in appropriate amounts. If you've got a dirty toxic bowel and you're eating the perfect diet, it will be completely wasted. Cleansing *must* take precedence, and a thorough bowel cleanse will take about a year, which includes the time you will need to rebuild the bowel with exercise and the right amount of appropriate nutrients.

Nearly all intestinal complaints are caused by poor eating habits. Processed foods turn into a sticky paste (egg white and flour make beautiful glues), and this adheres to the colon, forming layers of encrusted, ever-thickening mucus. It is said that if you ate just a teaspoon of this putrefying crust, it could kill you, and a really caked colon can weigh as much as 40 lbs! As digested food lumbers through what may only be a hole a pencil-width in thickness, it becomes very difficult for the body to draw nutriment from it, and anyone with a bowel in this state will only be using about ten per cent of their nutrition.

Ideally food should pass through the body completely every ten hours, yet it is not uncommon for people to retain faeces for days. To check how long your faeces are taking to pass through, try the sunflower seed test. Eat a really generous handful of seeds, chewing as little as possible. They'll be very evident when they emerge the other end, showing up white and grey in the faeces.

As the faeces stagnate and putrefy, the body is literally poisoned by the cesspool of decaying matter in its colon, first via the bloodstream and then into every cell in the body. This auto-intoxication is believed to be one of the sources of heart disorders, as a poisonous bloodstream raises serum cholesterol levels and predisposes the body to coronary disease. Tumours and cancer due to the biochemical changes associated with poor elimination are not uncommon, and of course such an overload increases the work of the other excretory organs, putting them under extra strain.

Laxatives

Nearly all laxatives are poisonous and irritant and do nothing to remove the encrusted mucus in the bowel. If they're used regularly, the colon becomes addicted to them and won't function without them, and as it grows weaker from overstimulation and irritation, the dose has to be gradually increased.

Diarrhoea

I hope those with chronic diarrhoea aren't thinking that at least all this isn't their problem. It may well be, because the cause of diarrhoea is a substance which irritates the colon so much that peristalsis goes into overdrive in an attempt to expel it. In some cases the build-up of old faeces trapped in the colon reaches such enormous proportions that these themselves induce rapid peristalsis, which is unceasing and results in chronic diarrhoea. In other words, you can be badly constipated and it will show itself as diarrhoea.

What is the ideal bowel movement?

1. Faeces should be buoyant when eliminated. Those that sink are heavy with mucus.
2. They should emerge easily and quickly and all of apiece within seconds of sitting down on the toilet, and as they float they should begin to break up. If it takes you more than five minutes to complete a bowel movement, you're constipated. One of my teachers used to joke that he knew how constipated strangers were by inspecting the amount of literature they kept in the toilet.
3. They should be a lightish brown in colour. If they emerge approximately the colour of the food you've been eating, for example, greenish-brown after lots of green vegetables, then you haven't digested the food properly. If they're yellow or chalky there's a problem with bile secretion or the production of digestive enzymes.
4. They should not smell noxious, though they will have a slight odour. If you go on a fruit fast for a week and the resultant faeces smell only of the fruit you've eaten, it's an excellent sign of a clean colon.
5. They should be four-fifths as bulky as the food you've eaten, and they should not be compacted.
6. They should emerge unaccompanied by gurgling, foaming, flatulence and general orchestration.

Dr Christopher's herbal combination to aid in proper bowel function

This is a superb formula for treating all bowel problems and is also helpful as part of the treatment for haemorrhoids. The combination of herbs cleanses the liver, the gall-bladder, starts the bile flowing, and stimulates the peristaltic muscle so that encrusted mucus will gradually be sloughed off and the bowel rebuilt, allowing food to be perfectly and properly assimilated.

1 part barberry bark (*Berberis vulgaris*)
2 parts cascara sagrada (*Rhamnus purshiana*)
1 part cayenne (*Capsicum annum*)
1 part goldenseal (*Hydrastis canadensis*)
1 part lobellia (*Lobelia inflata*)
1 part red raspberry leaves (*Rubus idaeus*)

1 part turkey rhubarb root (*Rheum palmatum*)
1 part ginger (*Zingiber officinale*)

Combine all the herbs, which should be finely powdered, and fill size '00' gelatin capsules with them (see page 129). Alternatively, you can mix 1¾ oz (49 g) into 144 pills (see page 130). You can buy these finely powdered herbs from the suppliers listed in the appendix and mix them up for yourself.

Dosage: begin by taking two capsules three times a day with meals. As there are no two people alike in age, size or physical constitution (and people's bowels are as variable as their fingerprints), you may well find you will have to regulate the dose according to your needs. If you get diarrhoea, cut down. If you can't get a bowel movement, then raise the dosage until you can. I know some of my patients have had to take as much as twelve or fourteen capsules with each meal. No matter. This is how it should be, because I must stress this formula is not a laxative. It is specifically designed to strip the bowel of accumulated mucus, detoxify and rebuild. Ideally you should have at least one bowel movement for every meal you eat.

The old bits of encrusted mucus that emerge may look very odd and range from nuts and seeds, which have been lodged in the colon for months or even years, traces of barium meal (if you've ever had one), bits of what looks like rubber tyre, tree bark, or coloured vaseline jelly. Don't be alarmed by any of this and do not taper off the formula so much that you lose momentum and continuity of this elimination. Keep it up for a minimum of six months. Most people need to do it for about nine months and some need to continue for a year. Combine this gastro-intestinal cleansing with a diet which is totally free of the mucus-forming foods: dairy products, eggs, meat and all refined processed foods. There's no point pulling out the mucus from one end and putting it in at the other. Expect, while following this course, that your faeces will smell stronger or fouler than usual, that they may look strange and vary considerably in colour from black to lumps which look like honey-coloured vaseline.

To determine when the process is at an end and your colon is perfectly clean, go on a carrot juice and purified water fast for a day, then watch your bowel movements. The faeces should emerge looking bright orange/brown. If they are a mixture of brown and orange/brown, then there is still old encrusted matter emerging and the cleansing needs to be continued. If they're completely brown, it means you've got a long way to go.

In the last few months of the bowel cleanse, taper down the dose gently and look to rebuilding the blood. There's no point in doing this sooner because the bloodstream will be too toxic to take full advantage of the herbs you're feeding it.

Rebuilding the blood

Take four size '00' capsules of finely powdered yellow dock, burdock and comfrey, equally mixed; three times daily with meals for two to three months. If you can't get powdered herbs, take two cups of herbal tea using three herbs daily. If you get diarrhoea, it means the colon is still in the process of eliminating all that encrusted mucus, so stop, wait until it has finished, and then try again. Tea and coffee are incompatible with iron-rich herbs, so don't drink them while taking this formula.

Also take three tablespoons of parsley juice every morning. You'll need a generous bunch to get this much juice. If you hate the taste, stir in another vegetable juice. To extract the juice, rinse the bunch of fresh parsley well under running water. Put it through a mincer – hand cranked or electric, it doesn't matter – then squeeze the pulped parsley in a muslin cloth, catching the juice in a basin. Keep any excess juice in the fridge; it will stay fresh for forty-eight hours. If you're lucky enough to have a juicer you can use this.

Take rejuvelac (see page 17) or plenty of live plain yoghurt during the first and last months of the cleansing to implant lots of friendly bacteria in the lower colon, and throughout the programme drink as much purified water as you can. By the time you're finished, you'll hopefully be addicted to pure water and will keep up this good habit.

Massage to help peristalsis

Do this throughout your bowel cleansing programme every morning. In many people poor diet has caused their peristaltic muscles to stop working altogether, and this simple massage will help to re-educate those lazy muscles. Peristalsis is simply the automatic wave-like movements of the alimentary canal by which food is propelled along it.

Lie on your back with your knees slightly bent and a cushion supporting your head and neck, as well as a cushion under your knees so the abdominal muscles are fully relaxed. Now envisage your lower colon. It comes up the right-hand side of the abdomen, crosses from right to left at about the level of your elbows when you hold your arms to your sides, and goes down the left-hand side of the abdomen. It is important you place it correctly in your mind's eye – you don't want to massage yourself from back to front. Begin deep down the left-hand side of the abdomen with *downward* pressure using the heel of your hand, and gradually work up the lower colon with pressure being exerted *downwards* all the time. Now turn the corner and work along the transverse colon23 pressing constantly to the left as you work your way along to the right. Turn the corner again and start on the ascending colon pressing *upwards* as you gradually work downwards.

Start again on the left-hand side of the abdomen and this time use a different type of massaging movement. Press your fingertips well into the abdomen using small circles in a clockwise direction. As you reach the *lowest* point of each circle, increase the pressure until it becomes almost a digging motion. Gradually work up the left-hand side of the abdomen, keeping up this movement until you reach the ribs. Now do the same to the transverse colon, passing from left to right in a line from elbow to elbow. Begin on the left with small clockwise circles and let the pressure at the end of each circle be a leftwards dig. Keep this up as you work your way to the right. Then press deeply with the heel of the hand from right to left along the route you've just come. Do this last heel-palm movement three times. Now go to work on the ascending colon with small circles where the main pressure is always *upward* while you gradually move down the right abdomen, pressing as deeply as possible. Then do three deep 'pull' strokes using the heel of your hand along the route you've just come.

Then move your hands to your navel and make small clockwise circles with your fingertips using plenty of pressure. Gradually move the circular movements outwards into a spiral, always following a clockwise direction. When the spiral reaches out to touch the lower colon, exert even more pressure with your finger tips. To finish, spread out your palm flat just beneath your navel and give the abdomen a good hard shaking. Relax. You'll need to, it is quite strenuous. Get up slowly. If anything hurts while doing this, ease up on the pressure a little, but ***don't give up on the exercise***. And don't be put off by lengthy instructions. It may sound complicated, but if you follow the instructions step by step you'll soon get the hang of it. Practice makes perfect and the results are worth the few minutes of daily effort.

The kidneys

One of my best teachers used to observe that he had never seen a healthy pair of kidneys, as observed in an iridology test, which is not surprising considering the amount of tea, coffee, cocoa, salt and other harmful substances with which we assault them daily. They are there to filter off impurities from the blood and balance the amount of salt and water retained by the body. They lie at the back wall of the abdomen right up near the ribs and, from the inner side of each kidney, a tube, the ureter, runs down the back of the abdominal cavity and enters the bladder. When it exits, it is called the urethra, and its opening is in front of the vagina in women and at the tip of the penis in men. In women it is quite short, which tends to mean they are more prone to cystitis than men because bacteria will invade this short length more easily.

The greatest proportion of our bodies is water. About one gallon of water is eliminated daily through the skin, the kidneys and other eliminative organs. It is obviously vital to have an exact mechanism for controlling overall body water content. Doubly so because even a tiny increase of water in the bloodstream leads to a disproportionate increase in blood pressure. Chemical diruetics are mainly prescribed to reduce blood pressure because, if the water content of the body can be made to dwindle by as little as two per cent, the systolic reading can drop by anything between twenty to thirty points. But these chemicals work by irritating the delicate tubules in the kidneys and forcing them to pass more water. Besides which, they leach potassium from the body to such an extent that synthetic potassium has to be given, and that begins the 'knock-on' effect or allopathic medicine, where one drug has to be prescribed to offset the side-effects of the first.

In herbal medicine diuretics are used to treat infections of the urinary tract like cystitis, to help with water retention, obesity, nerve inflammations which may be connected with the improper workings of the kidneys like lumbago and sciatica, skin complaints, kidney stones and lymphatic swellings. The beauty of herbs is that they're all rich in potassium. Some of them do irritate the kidneys, so it is always safest to counteract this by administering them with a demulcent – that is, herbs which are rich in mucilage and so have softening, protective and soothing actions taken internally – like comfrey, marshmallow, slippery elm or fenugreek in proportions of twenty per cent demulcent to eighty per cent diuretic. Good diuretics include agrimony, almonds, ash, burdock, buchu, birch, broom, blackcurrant leaves, bramble, briar, cleavers, conchgrass, dog's tooth (*Cynodon dactylon*), dandelion, hawthorn, heather, horsetail, juniper, maize tassels, marshmallow, meadow-sweet, nettles, parsley, plaintain, pellitory of the wall, rose, summer savoury, sage, uva-ursi, strawberry, raspberry, and redcurrant leaves. If you suffer from hay fever, don't take pellitory of the wall – it may lead to allergic rhinitus. Cleavers should not be used by diabetics.

It is inadvisable to treat yourself for a urinary infection or kidney stones without first seeking the advice of a medical herbalist, as clumsy self-help might make the situation worse. But you can make a good start by drinking lots of purified water, potassium-rich broths (see page 102) and fruit juices, avoiding tea, coffee, cocoa and salt absolutely, and concentrating on a diet rich in fresh fruit and vegetables, low in animal products and free of all processed foods. Strawberries are particularly helpful as they help to dispel uric acid, and the only vegetables and fruit to avoid are spinach and rhubarb which contain large quantities of oxalic acid. However, if the kidneys are weak, it is not advisable to drink gallons of water as this will only aggravate the already overburdened organs. You can tell if you have waterlogged kidneys if you have dark circles under your eyes, or if they're very baggy. In which case take a herbal diuretic. A gentle diuretic can be made by mixing 1 oz (28 g) of anise seed with 2 oz (56 g) each of dried melon and cucumber seeds. Grind them in a meat mincer. Mix with honey and eat one teaspoon with each meal.

Yearly kidney cleanse

Once a year it is an excellent idea to go on a three-day kidney cleansing fast. Choose May, when asparagus tips are just coming through. Buy a large bunch and mince the raw green tips, catching the juice in a bowl. Take a tablespoon of this juice every four hours. Drink nothing but purified water and take one pint of the following tea daily divided into three portions:

> 4 oz (112 g) dandelion root (*Taraxacum officinale*)
> 4 oz (112 g) horsetail herb (*Equisetum arvense*)
> 2 oz (56 g) comfrey root (*Symphytum officinale*)
> 1 oz (28 g) cinnamon (*Cinnamomum zeylanicum*)

Make a decoction of 1 oz to 1 pint. It may be drunk hot or cold. Once you've finished the asparagus juice, go on with the tea for eight more days until it is finished. Daily apply a hot ginger root compress over the kidneys while you're on your three-day fast. Leave on for half an hour (see directions for compresses page 132).

The skin

The skin is a two-way street: it flushes outwards and ingests inwards. It's your body's largest eliminative organ, and when healthy excretes one-third of your body's waste. Think of it as your third kidney. Its hundreds of thousands of sweat glands not only regulate the body's temperature, but also act as miniature kidneys, detoxifying organs and working to cleanse the blood and free the system from suffocating poisons. Indeed, sweat contains nearly the same constituents as urine. If the skin becomes lazy, its pores get choked up with millions of dead cells and uric acid, and other rubbish gets trapped in the body so that the liver and kidneys have to work extra hard to carry their added burdens. Eventually they in turn can't stand the strain, and start to break down and dump poisons and waste in the tissues.

We ought to shed at least a pound of waste products daily through the skin, but most of us manage only a paltry few ounces. As well as its eliminative work, skin actually breathes, absorbing oxygen and exhaling carbon dioxide formed in the tissues. We are capable of absorbing certain nutrients through the skin, like sea water and sea air, and of course we manufacture our own vitamin D by exposing the skin to a reasonable degree of sunshine.

How to help your skin

1.   Profuse sweating from regular exercise. Turkish baths and saunas help too. Neither should be taken if you have high blood pressure.

2.   Wear only natural fabrics next to the skin. Synthetics suffocate it. Make sure your underwear and your clothes consist only, ideally, of cotton, or failing that, linen, silk or wool. Your feet and hands are particularly richly endowed with sweat glands, so don't cheat on these areas by wearing nylon socks and non-leather shoes.

3.   Use only organic soaps to wash with. Soap made from olive oil is excellent and Molo and Weleda make good ones. Don't go mad on the soap. It is only necessary to wash areas which sweat or get dirty – armpits, genitals, under the breast, hands and feet.

4.   Use natural oils on the skin like almond, olive or avocado, not mineral oils or other synthetics like baby oil which is made from petrol.

5.   Help the skin to eliminate by dry brushing daily.

The benefits of dry skin brushing

1.   It will effectively remove the dead layers of skin and other impurities so that the pores are open and eliminating without obstruction.

2.   It stimulates circulation, so that the blood nourishes those organs of the body which lie near the surface particularly effectively.

3.   It assists and increases the eliminative capacity of the skin.

4.   It stimulates the hormone- and oil-producing glands.

5.   It has a wonderfully powerful rejuvenating effect on the nervous system by stimulating nerve endings in the skin, and for this reason is particularly beneficial for people who feel sluggish or depressed.

6.   It helps to stop colds when used in combination with a hot/cold shower.

7.   It builds up healthier muscle tone and a better distribution of fat deposits, getting rid of unsightly lumps and bumps. Five minutes of energetic scrubbing is the equivalent of

thirty minutes of jogging or other physical exercise as far as body tone is concerned.

8. It is a highly effective technique for stimulating the expulsion of any fresh lymphatic mucus or hardened or impacted lymph nodes. If you couple it with a colon cleanse, you will see the lymph mucoid appearing in the stools, looking like vaseline, feeling jelly-like, and ranging from practically clear to dark brown.

9. It helps to prevent premature ageing and gives you a terrific sense of well-being. I've never yet encountered a patient of mine who didn't love it once they got used to it.

How to skin brush

You must use a **natural** bristle brush with a long handle. The ones I import are made of Mexican tampico fibre which does not gouge and scratch the skin. Sainsburys also sell a good one. **Nylon and synthetic fibre won't do**, nor will loofahs or hand mitts. (It takes 20-30 minutes of loofah scrubbing daily to get the effect you can achieve with just five minutes of skin scrubbing).

Start with the soles of your feet and a dry body. Vigorously pass the dry brush over every skin surface except the face and genital area. Avoid the nipples too if they're sensitive. Use clean, upward-sweeping strokes, not rotary, scrubbing or back-and-forth motions. Everything below the heart should be upwards, and everything above downwards. You can brush across the top of the shoulders and upper back for better skin contact, unless you can entice your nearest and dearest into the bathroom to do it for you. Pay particular attention to the soles of your feet and the palms of your hands which are packed with nerve endings and will benefit particularly from brushing.

Begin with light pressure until your skin gets used to it, then increase it. Brush until your skin gets rosy and glows. Do this at least once daily on rising for five minutes. You can also repeat it at night, but not too near bedtime or you won't sleep.

Brush every day for three months, then brush two or three days weekly. Skin brushing is subject, as are herbs, to homeostatic resistance, that is, your skin will get used to it and stop responding so well.

Don't brush skin that is irritated, damaged or infected. Go round it. Don't let the rest of the family share your brush, for obvious hygienic reasons. Treat your brush as if it was your personal toothbrush. Brush the scalp to stimulate hair growth and free the scalp of dandruff and other impurities. If your hair is very long you may prefer to massage the scalp with the flat of the fingertips, using an action which actually *moves* the scalp skin, not a shampooing action. Work from the back of the scalp towards the eyebrows.

Showering

After a brush, remove the dead skin cells by showering or rubbing down with a sponge. Take a hot shower or bath using an organic soap, then take a hot shower for three minutes followed by a cold one for twenty seconds. Revert to the hot shower and then the cold, extending the time of the latter. Move the shower head from your feet upwards, and finish by holding it over the medulla oblongata at the base of the skull, letting the cold water run from there down your spine. When you start breathing hard, this means your body has had sufficient. This hot/cold technique will alkalinise the blood, clear the head, and has a very beneficial effect on the vital functions of the body, especially on the glandular system.

Wash your brush in warm, soapy water using a natural soap once weekly. Rinse it well under cool running water, then towel it dry and leave it in the airing cupboard to dry out completely.

Herbs which help the skin are those which purify and build the blood and support the kidneys. Diaphoretics to induce sweating can also be used, **but only with discrimination and caution** as they are not appropriate for many conditions. A gentle diaphoretic may be taken by drinking medicinal teas of catnip or lemon balm, and by taking hand or foot baths of the same. These will soothe the skin and get it working properly again. More powerful diaphoretics like elderflowers, yarrow, peppermint, cayenne, ginger boneset, hyssop, blessed thistle, and mustard are used to 'sweat out' an illness like a cold or a fever.

The lymphatic system

This is best described as the body's vacuum system. It doesn't have a pump like a heart, but it moves the lymphatic fluids round the body with muscle and lung motion through a one-way valve system, picking up poisons as it goes and dumping them in the waste stations called lymph glands situated in the groin, behind the knees, in the armpits, and under the chin. A network of tubes about the diameter of a needle carrying lymph fluid penetrates the remotest nooks and crannies of the body, covering every area except the central nervous system. These lymph vessels are populated by billions of white blood cells all hungrily bent on attacking and ingesting invaders and cleaning up debris. Each one has a specialised role: some hunt for foreign invading cells, while others form antibodies which immobilise the invader when it comes.

The red blood system's main organ is, of course, the heart. The lymph system (which you can loosely think of as the white blood system) looks to the thymus gland, which is found beneath the breastbone just above the heart. During childhood the thymus instructs white cells to make antibodies, and has the wonderful ability of recognising which cell is part of you and which isn't. So it programmes the way the immune system works, making sure that this system doesn't turn its activities against the body's own tissues.

If the thymus breaks down you become prey not only to infection but to cancer and auto-immune diseases. When the lymph system breaks down in women it is particularly significant, because it is generally the lymphatic nodules which give women the lump problems under the arms, on the shoulders and in the breast. Leap to attention if your lymph glands swell up. It means your lymph system is poisonous and needs help quickly.

The importance of exercise

Remember the lymph fluid is propelled round the body by both voluntary and involuntary muscular action. The best way to get your lymph system moving is by trampolining gently, and several companies are now producing a small, three or four foot diameter trampoline for use in the home. If you think you're fragile or if you're elderly, it's best to start trampolining under the supervisory eye of a trained instructor in a gym. If you're reasonably fit you can begin with the following exercises:

1. Keeping your arms and shoulders relaxed, gradually start bouncing up and down on your trampoline, breathing in deeply and exhaling completely with each bounce.
2. Now put your arms out parallel to your shoulders and, as

you continue to bounce, move your arms in a circular motion, beginning with small tight circles and expanding them to bigger ones until you're moving your arms as if you were holding a skipping rope.

3. Slow down to a steady jog, raising your knees so your feet are four inches off the trampoline, but don't keep this up for too long. It's pretty strenuous. If it proves too much in the beginning, simply walk on the trampoline, lifting your knees a little.

4. Go back to a steady bouncing and shuffle your feet back and forth in mid-air, first one foot, then the other.

5. Now twist your body from the waist down as you bounce, first to one side, then the other. It helps to steady yourself by holding your arms out.

6. Finally, a very energetic exercise. While bouncing, kick one foot out in front of you, lifting it as high as you can. Do the other side alternately.

A ten-minute daily bounce will really get your lymph system going. Failing that, take up swimming, lots of long, steady laps, and strong arm and leg movements, or jogging if you're very strong, preferably on soft surfaces like grass. Cement or hard surfaces can be very shocking to your organs and intestines if your muscle tone is poor.

Skin brushing is a superb way to move the lymph round the body, but it should not be done instead of, but rather as well as, exercise. You may notice when you begin your skin brushing that a lot of lymph mucus appears in the faeces initially.

Lymph-cleansing herbs

Cleansing the lymph system will take several months, as hardened or thickened lymph mucus is broken down and flushed away. The most effective herbs for this are echinacea, iceberg lettuce, goldenseal, myrrh and bayberry bark. As the lymph is being cleansed, a lot of poisons will be thrown off into the bloodstream, so it is always best to combine a lymph-cleansing herb with one which will also cleanse the blood. Happily, echinacea, which is the finest lymph cleanser in the herbal kingdom, is also an excellent blood cleanser. It actually helps to encourage the production of white blood cells.

A good general lymph-cleansing formulation is:

2 parts echinacea (*Echinacea angustifolia*)
1 part red clover (*Trifolium pratense*)
1 part bayberry bark (*Myrica cerifera*)
1 part lobelia (*Lobelia inflata*)
1 part plantain (*Plantago spp*)

Take two size '00' capsules three times daily with meals for a maximum of eight months.

The lungs

Our lungs never stop moving. We can live without food for several months, without water for several days, but we cannot live without air for even a few minutes. In order to ensure its intake, the chest muscles and diaphragm work together like bellows, squeezing the lungs regularly so that air is forced in and out through the windpipe to keep up a fresh supply of oxygen. These movements are automatically controlled by a little pacemaker at the base of the brain called the medulla oblongata. Its task is to send regular messages to the muscles of the chest and diaphragm telling them to squeeze and relax their grip on the lungs. It benefits greatly from a massage with a forceful cold shower held over it so that the water is left to run down the spine.

When at rest we breathe about twelve times a minute. If you need extra oxygen, as when you're running, your breathing increases to double or even treble that rate. The problem is most of us are sloppy breathers. We use only the top third of the lungs and exacerbate the problem by slouching.

How to breathe properly

Improve your posture by standing and sitting tall and lying so that you're well stretched out. Keep your head well up and don't tuck your chin in or let it jut out. Check your posture by standing barefoot against a wall without a skirting board. Try to flatten the whole length of your spine against the wall, keeping the back of your head against it too. Now stretch up and exhale deeply. Walk away from the wall holding this position and remember this is how you should always stand and walk.

For those with breathing problems, brisk, sustained walking with plenty of short rests is the best type of exercise. Consciously work to control your lung capacity by breathing in while you walk four paces, holding for a further four steps (don't explode – if it feels uncomfortable, let it go), then breathing out slowly with control for six paces. As you get better, increase the count proportionately.

Swimming gently and consistently is also recommended. Shower off all the chlorine meticulously afterwards.

Check the quality of the air you breathe. Is it full of other people's smoke? If so, object! Avoid damp, cold or foggy air and extreme temperatures. If you can, avoid areas with a high pollen count and polluted air in the heart of cities where the poisons are dangerously high. Use an ioniser to correct the balance of the ions in the air, that is, the tiny electric particles flowing in the air around you, particularly in your bedroom, where you spend at least eight hours out of every twenty-four, in your car and your office. You can leave windows open or closed while they're in use. Either way, they'll cope. Positive ionisers are best, but negative ones will do. (For suppliers see the appendix.)

Breathing exercises

1.   Lie flat on the floor, your head and neck cushioned by a pillow and your knees comfortably bent and supported by another pillow underneath. Check that there are no disturbing draughts. Place one hand on the abdomen just below the navel, and now breathe in and make it rise. Breathe out and feel it fall as you imagine sinking deeper and deeper into the floor. ***Don't move your chest***. Now breathe in to a mental count of four as the stomach rises, hold your breath to a count of four and breathe out to a count of eight, controlling exhalation slowly as the stomach sinks. As the diaphragm gets stronger, increase the exhalation count. Do this for a few minutes every day. (Asthmatics will find this kind of exercise particularly good to help control attacks.)

2.   Push your bottom well back into a hard chair, feet flat on the floor, sit up straight and put your fintertips just level with the inner margin of the ribs where left and right diverge. Let the head, shoulders and chest slump forward. Breathe in with control, straightening up. Now breathe out, slumping forward, pressing the air out with the hands

as long as you feel comfortable. Repeat six times and don't hold your breath in between.

Don't block up your lungs with catarrh-forming foods: dairy products, eggs, meat, sugar, tea, coffee, chocolate and all refined foods. Put plenty of garlic and onions in your diet, raw if at all possible, as neither are as effective if cooked. Alternatively, use oil or syrup of garlic. Massage blocked or inflamed sinuses with fresh lemon juice externally, rubbing it into the skin. They can also be helped by chewing freshly grated horseradish root macerated in cider vinegar. Chew a teaspoon after every meal and when you're grating it breathe in the fumes as deeply as you can. Have a box of tissues standing by because it will flush out blocked sinuses very effectively.

Herbal steam bath to decongest and strengthen the lungs

Mix one ounce of wormwood and eucalyptus together in equal proportions. Put into a basin and pour over two pints of boiling water. Crush two cloves of garlic and add. Stir well. Measure in five drops of sage oil. Cover the head with a towel and hold the face eight inches away from the infusion. Keep the eyes closed and breathe in and out steadily through the nose, keeping the mouth closed. Do this for twenty minutes if you can manage it, and do it three times a day. You may use the same mixture three times over, but add freshly crushed garlic each time.

Herbs which strengthen and help the lungs are mullein, comfrey, sweet marjoram, elecampagne, lobelia, valerian, ginseng, German camomile, eucalyptus, myrrh, coltsfoot, hyssop, angelica, elderberries, rosemary, ground ivy, horehound, Irish moss, liquorice, vervain, Icelandic moss, thyme, marshmallow, lungwort, grindelia, sage, and of course garlic. Best to use mild herbs like sage, comfrey and mullein in daily herbal teas as a prophylactic, and to take lots of onions, horseradish and garlic daily in the diet, saving the rest to treat coughs, colds, and other lung problems as specifically needed. Some herbs like coltsfoot, rosemary and mullein can be smoked to relieve bronchial congestion, but this must be supervised by a medical herbalist. Others can be applied over the lungs in poultice or fomentation form, taken as oils in honey a few drops at a time, or taken powdered as snuff.

Any healthy person will benefit from a deep cleansing of the five eliminative channels to raise them to peak fitness. It's a good way to begin a new lifestyle of reformed diet, exercise, relaxation, and attitude. Those who are sick need additional herbs to help the affected parts, something to balance the glands or to help the liver and gall-bladder, for example. You may then begin to feel you're rattling with gelatin capsules, but do remember you can help yourself with herbs other than orally, by their external application in baths, oils, fomentations, poultices, herbal steams, enemas, douches, pessaries, smoking and snuffs. I should stress it is not how many herbs you use but the way in which a few herbs can be successfully administered which is the secret of successful herbalism.

Cleansing reactions

To understand why you may get cleansing reactions during the course of natural treatment, it is first necessary to understand how allopathy, or modern chemical medicine works. An allopathic remedy will try and counteract the symptoms of an illness, so that if you're feverish the doctor will give you a chemical remedy to bring down the fever, or surgically remove an organ which is malfunctioning and is debilitated, or suppress a pain with pain killers. A medical herbalist will not suppress symptoms, but will give a remedy to move the toxic substances causing the illness out of the body and, having done this, will set to work on strengthening and balancing the system. As these toxins are moved out, the body will show cleansing reactions: aches and general discomfort, dizziness, itching, nausea, skin or bowel upsets, or, interestingly, the symptoms of disease from the most recent to those going right back to childhood.

If all this worries you, let me say this: cleansing reactions can be vastly modified by careful management following two simple steps:

1.   Keep all your channels of elimination, the major and minor ones, open and working freely, but keep your cleansing within manageable limits. By which I mean don't go at your new health programme like a bull at a gate. Alter your life in well-managed steps. By all means give

up tea, coffee, salt, anything processed or refined, meat, eggs, dairy products, but **not all at once** unless you're critically ill, otherwise you'll experience an enormous cleansing reaction. And three cups of medicinal herbal tea is **not** better for you if I have stated only one.

2.   Fast one day weekly on a regular basis if you're a subject suited to fasting (see the following section on fasting).

If your cleansing reaction is still intolerably vigorous, you'll need to see a medical herbalist who will have the experience to alter your formulation by carefully selecting various herbs to steady and rebalance your system. This is quite a complex and delicate process and outside the range of self-treatment.

If you want to get off to a really good start to a general eliminative programme, go on a fast to decoke the body rapidly. It is better to fast for one day a week on a regular basis than for two consecutive weeks a year, because little, regular and often is far preferable to one big strenuous bang as far as the stabilisation and maintenance of your health is concerned.

Why fast?

Fasting is a marvellous way to accelerate the healing process because it literally incinerates years of accumulated rubbish in the system, throwing it out through every available orifice. The digestive process takes up thirty per cent of the total energy of the body, so if it is placed in a complete state of rest, it can concentrate entirely on the matter in hand – detoxification and healing.

Sick animals don't eat, and feverish little children left to their own devices will refuse food and ask only for fresh fruit juices (as long as their digestions haven't been corrupted by squashes or fizzy drinks). So fasting can be used both to assist the healing process and as preventative medicine, to maintain the body at peak fitness when well by shedding accumulated poisons and preparing the body to utilise nutrition far more efficiently once the fast is broken.

It should be remembered that the body doesn't just rid itself of poor nutritional waste, but sloughs off the toxic effects of stress, grief and anger which often have more to do with the foundation of illness than any other factor.

How to fast

Fasting on purified water alone is not only a miserable experience for bodies heavy with toxins, but the particularly nasty ones, the result of ingesting insecticides and poisonous metals, gush into the system so fast that they can induce self-poisoning. It is much better to drink alkaline juices, not only because they soften the initial vigorous side-effects of fasting, but also because the healing process is actually accelerated by the ingestion of a superabundance of vitamins, minerals and enzymes, and fruit juices maintain a stable electrolyte balance, ensuring the circulation remains steady, while water alone has the dangerous capacity to distort it.

The day before a fast, eat only light meals, concentrating particularly on raw fruit and vegetables. Drink two cups of slippery elm gruel, sweetened with a little honey and flavoured with a pinch of cinnamon, during the course of the day. This will soothe any irritability in the gastro-intestinal tract and prepare it for the fast.

On rising

Skin scrub vigorously so that waste from the lymph can be moved into the bowel (see page 154), then take an enema (see page 133). If you simply can't face an enema, use a good dose of bowel tonic instead and begin your fast with two 8 oz glasses of prune juice, but an enema is more effective. The herb you choose for your enema depends on your reason for fasting. If you're sick and feverish, then catnip or camomile are both excellent for soothing and calming the body. If you are weak and emaciated, slippery elm will nourish and soothe an inflamed or weak bowel.

Coffee enemas are popular, because they are readily absorbed into the lining of the colon travelling up the haemorrhoidal vein to stimulate the gall-bladder and liver, causing them to dump their contents quickly without unduly straining other organs. The enema should be made with freshly ground coffee, one ounce to one pint, and injected at body temperature. However, I find chicory root far more effective and it does not have the stimulating side-effect that coffee does. It is more effective for people with constipation, persistent biliousness due to an overstrained liver, and is useful for gout and rheumatic complaints. Besides which it is cheaper. Use a standard decoction and inject at body temperature.

A good general herbal detoxifying enema mixture is agrimony, yellow dock and burdock in equal quantities made as a standard decoction. Spirulina plankton enemas are good for those whose energy is very low and it also acts as an appetite suppressant, useful for those who can't ignore the hunger pangs while fasting. However, it is **not** recommended for people with lymph congestion, because it works by dumping toxins from the body's tissues directly into the lymphatic system, and the result can be painful joints and an even more overburdened lymphatic system.

Having selected and taken your enema, take only fruit juices, preferably freshly pressed, and purified water for the rest of the day and evening. There's no limit to how much you can drink. If you feel faint, drink a hot herbal tea with a teaspoonful of honey or hot diluted cider vinegar, honey and water. Make sure you drink something at least every two hours, even if you don't feel like it. Stick to one type of fruit juice, don't mix it. Any kind is acceptable but its better to drink fruit juice which is not imported. So apple and pear juice would be more suitable for British constitutions, while orange juice would suit Californians and grape juice would work better for Mediterranean people. Fruit juices are more aggressive cleansers than vegetable juices. You are allowed to mix vegetable juices – tomato and carrot, spinach and beetroot, and add some pressed herb juice. My fast day is my favourite day of the week. I consider it pure self-indulgence because for once I can concentrate totally on nurturing myself. This nurturing has its spiritual dimensions too, so don't watch television, which is too stimulating; listen to a favourite record instead. Read, go for a walk, sit outside and sunbathe for half an hour. Above all, relax and, while you do so, do some deep breathing exercises. Let your body enjoy its natural rhythm.

If you are only able to rest once during the day, make it midday. By lying down you increase the flow of blood to the liver, which is valiantly carrying out its detoxifying work, by forty per cent. If you apply heat to the liver and stomach area, this flow is increased by at least another twenty per cent. So place a hot water bottle on your stomach, or better still, wrap yourself from ribcage to groin in a steaming hot towel, then put a plastic bin bag round you to save dripping all over the sheets and retire to bed for an hour well covered in blankets.

If for any reasons you get stomach cramps, sip peppermint or camomile tea and use the hot water bottle routine. Avoid hot baths, saunas, strenuous activity, driving, or too much reading because you may find your eyesight isn't as sharp as usual. Certainly don't smoke.

Preparing for sleep

On the night of the fast, you'll probably find you need less sleep than usual. Go to bed with a quiet mind and warm feet. If your body temperature drops, which is not at all unusual while fasting, take a mustard foot bath before bed and sip a cup of lemon balm tea.

Sleep with a window open. You'll need as much oxygen as possible, so don't suffocate yourself with central heating. If you're cold, use extra blankets. If you still can't sleep, get up and run a warm bath. Add a muslin bag full of camomile to the water and, while relaxing in the bath, rub yourself all over with it.

Breaking the fast

George Bernard Shaw said, 'Any fool can go on a fast, but it takes a wise man to break it properly.' If you rush into a heavy breakfast the next day, you'll overload your unprepared stomach. So break your fast by slowly chewing a ripe apple. For lunch, eat lightly baked or steamed vegetables or fruit (not both). For supper have soupy grains like lentils, millet or buckwheat. This is especially important if you've chosen to fast for more than one day. If you've fasted for more than a week, the 'break-in' period should be extended to three days and so on in proportion.

Who should not fast?

The very elderly, fragile or emaciated.

Those with weak hearts.

Those who are mentally ill.

Pregnant women.

Those with physically very active careers like weight-lifting instructors.

Those with TB.

Those with diabetes. Hypoglycaemics may fast, but they must also take 500 mg B_6 and 1 B complex while doing so.

Those who are dubious about fasting or fail to understand its benefits even after explanation, because they will almost certainly fail and get trapped in a depressing spiral of negative thinking.

I have known all of these groups, except the last, to benefit from fasts, but they must be supervised by qualified medical herbalists, nutritionists or naturopaths who are really experienced in this field.

Side-effects

The body will use all the eliminative channels, major or minor, to excrete waste. Your body odour may change and get quite rank or salty, so skin scrubbing and bathing is especially important, and don't block the pores with oils, deodorants or lotions. Your tongue will get furry. Use a toothbrush to scrub it, **not** an antiseptic mouthwash. You may produce more ear wax than usual, get dandruff, spots, produce a lot of phlegm, get a headache, feel cold and shivery. In which case take things gently, wrap up, spit out the phlegm into a handkerchief or tissue, don't swallow it; use cotton wool buds to cleanse the wax; do your deep breathing exercises.

On the other hand you may get none of these side-effects, in which case don't be disappointed and think the fast is not working. It is, so persist. It simply means that you're less overburdened with waste than most, or that your body is off-loading toxins through another more comfortable channel which you may not readily notice, like your kidneys.

You will not feel at all sexually active during the course of a fast, particularly a short one, but after finishing it you may well feel sexually rejuvenated. Many of my patients have been surprised at how enthusiastic they've felt about sex after a three or four day or even longer fast.

A good cleanse using all the eliminative channels and a three day fast, followed by regular weekly fasting, is a wonderful way to ensure and improve your health. It is the sort of treatment that can easily be carried out in your own home and the benefits you'll reap will clear up your skin, strengthen your hair and your nails, help you reach your ideal body weight, put a sparkle in your eye and a spring in your step. Besides all the obvious and visible effects, a deep cleanse will ensure the healthy function of all your internal organs, ridding you of problems like flatulence, indigestion, constipation, breathlessness and swollen glands, and it will raise your whole level of well-being to a vibrant pitch you may have felt was impossible to achieve.

A one day weekly rest from food will accelerate the action of the herbs, but if you simply can't fast don't worry. The herbs will still have an excellent effect only they will work more slowly. Consistency is the vital pre-requisite to successful herbal treatment. So begin now and persist. Make this the year you finally become truly healthy.

CHAPTER 6

Stress:
The Root of Illness

Getting ill is never accidental. We become ill because our bodies are trying to teach us something, and we ignore the lesson at our peril. If we don't adjust our diet, our habits, re-examine our emotional and spiritual attitudes, we are liable to get sicker later on. People tend to feel very negative about illness. I try to encourage my patients to look on the positive side of any illness, to see it as an opportunity not just for struggle and pain, but for enlightenment and growth, as an ideal means to build on strengths and understand weaknesses. I've seen people get ill because it was the only way they could ask for love and involvement. I've had patients hang onto their illness because they were afraid to get better, or because they used their illness as a brickbat or a 'bribe' for their nearest and dearest, or as a means of punishing themselves for past failings. Above all, I've seen an enormous number of people succumb to illness because of stress.

Depression

The mentally ill occupy more than a third of all NHS beds. Our society seems to be driving people mad on an unprecedented scale. Giving people tranquillisers merely attacks the symptoms. It does nothing to change the cause of the suffering. Factors which increase the likelihood of depression are isolation, not having a close confidant, not going out to work, bad housing and financial problems, looking after toddlers at home full time and losing your mother when you were a child.

Yet depression can be greatly alleviated by purposeful activity. Samuel Johnson, who was a depressive, found action was the key to triumphing over it. Such action didn't, in his opinion, necessarily have to be strenuous. He recommended 'chemistry, or a course of rope dancing, or a course of anything'. The main thing was participating, risking, daring, doing. It's not lack of ability which results in life's failures. It's lack of courage. So get out and get involved. Don't get hidebound with routine. Don't give up. Take plenty of daily exercise and make sure it's something you enjoy. Say what you mean. Don't be afraid to show your feelings. Don't procrastinate. Enjoy the pleasure of achievement. When working with depressives I find it necessary to point out that we are *all* vulnerable, physically and mentally, otherwise they tend to hang onto their pain and loneliness like some sort of secret talisman, behaving as if their condition were unique. Society considers vulnerability a weakness and covers it up with a show of strength. Depressives have to realise that our strength comes from our ability to acknowledge, to respect that vulnerability and be taught the difference between respect and indulgence. I think education of the emotions will be our most important aspect of health education over the next century.

Combatting stress

Modern society certainly does not have a monopoly on stress, or for that matter alcoholism or drug addiction. Old herbals bulge with prescriptions intended to combat 'spleene, melancholie, frantiquines, trubelisum sleep, the mare and the nag'. It's just that we've become more aware of the fundamental role stress plays in so much illness. Certainly we all need a little of it to keep us on our toes, and without it we'd atrophy emotionally and suffocate in our own inertia. The question is how much and for how long? Everyone's stress level is both different and variable. What is severely stressful to me may be no more than a niggling incident to you.

Negative attitudes and stress

Much depends on how much negativity you saddle yourself with – fear, hate, fury, wrath, bitterness, jealousy and anger. Other people don't make you feel these emotions; you make yourself feel them. So you can make yourself not feel them. Such control requires a lot of discipline and self-examination, but the end result, serenity and health, is worth the struggle!

Begin by examining some of your most fundamental attitudes. I used to indulge in a lot of self-righteous histrionics until I finally realised there's no such thing as righteous anger, simply because everyone, no matter how appalling I might think they were, had a right to be wrong. Including myself. So now if people hurt me, I know there's no point in getting righteously angry over their silliness; nor is there any profit in allowing them to manipulate me.

It may sound corny, but I've always found the old adage of counting from one to ten a good way of cooling off. Words spilled in anger are twice as difficult to erase afterwards. It also helps to tackle a difficult task immediately, no matter how painful or tedious it may be. I constantly remind myself how much getting upset is hurting me, and it saves me sloping off into all those stress-induced diseases ranging from hypertension to asthma to coronary thrombosis.

Priorities

It's easy to get things out of perspective if you worry too much, and as I was one of the world's great worriers I speak from experience. Notice the past tense. I learned to stop doing it. One of the things that sobered me up was the simple realisation that, if you placed every single member of the world's two thousand million inhabitants shoulder to shoulder on the Isle of Wight, you'd still have room for more. That thought gave me a sense of perspective about my own insignificance in a universal context. Matched against the infinite world of nature, my own anxieties seemed trivial.

I also learned to accept that life is full of uncertainties and that there are things which are truly beyond my control. So I simply have to stop trying to alter them. Standing back gives one a better view.

One of my saving graces has always been the importance I place on my family and friends. People seem to overvalue outside relationships and priorities centred round work, career, and hobbies, and undervalue the relationships with those they can really achieve something with directly and personally – family and friends. I've found that support from those you love is the single most important protection against the effects of stress.

Stress response

Humans react to stress in much the same way as animals do. There's an instant change in the muscles and organs of the body as it prepares for fight or flight. Heart-rate increases, blood pressure rockets, pupils dilate, blood flow into the muscles increases, while blood flow to the skin and digestive tract decreases. The bronchi expand so that the lungs can draw in more air, and the adrenalin pumping out from the adrenals mobilises energy reserves in the liver and muscles, making glucose immediately available for energy demands. At this stage, the body is on·red alert, ready to fight or run. When the threat ends, these reactions are reversed. Alternatively, we learn to adapt to a stimulus that originally put the body into this state of fight or flight, so that someone living near Heathrow, for example, becomes relatively untroubled by the roar of aircraft.

Physical reactions to stress may include tiredness, weakness, sweating, trembling, breathlessness, choking, fainting, hyperventilation, palpitation, digestive upsets. Or it may show itself as an overdependence òn alcohol, drugs or tobacco, loss of interest in sex, insomnia, or simply a succession of mysterious aches and pains and niggling little discomforts.

Relaxing

It is pointless telling someone to relax when they simply don't know how to. Yet relaxation is possible to learn, just as it is possible to learn to read or ride a bike. The choice of methods is wide and not all methods are suitable for every person. Meditation, yoga, self-hypnosis, visualisation, autogenics, biofeedback; keep trying until you settle on a method that's right for you. Don't be discouraged that you're not instantly brilliant at it. After all, could you learn to play a musical instrument in a week? The secret is to find a method you like and to persist with it.

The following herbs are listed individually and, unless otherwise stated, should be used singly as part of an overall cleansing treatment. You'd be surprised how often your repetitive headaches are the result of a blocked bowel or your lethargic depression the result of a sluggish lymph system. So an overall cleanse is a must. Besides which, moods are as variable as the people who get them and happily nature provides a large variety of herbs which each work, elegantly and subtly, on particular emotions. I wouldn't, for example, use powerful scullcap on a fractious baby, because it copes with more serious adult problems like drug addiction and alcoholism as well as high blood pressure and nervous headaches. Instead I'd go for camomile which I'd also use on myself if I'd eaten too much and was regretting it.

So read the following list of herbs and choose one that suits your condition. Having done so, stay with it. Remember herbs help slowly.

Camomile (*Matricaria chamomilla*)

There are two well-known camomiles: German camomile, as above, and common camomile, *Anthemis nobilis*, and at least fifty species of the genus scattered throughout the world. *Anthemis nobilis* can easily be distinguished from its chief rival because it is nearly prostrate, only 10-30 cm tall compared to the 60 cm achieved by the other.

Both have approximately the same medicinal properties, helping to soothe and calm the nervous system, relieve biliousness and flatulence, and help with the type of headaches some women get before a period. *Matricaria* is particularly effective for the kind of throbbing headaches that make one restless and irritable.

Make an infusion using half an ounce of the dried flowers to one pint of water, remembering to cover it instantly, because much of its healing properties are in the azulene which will escape through vaporisation. Brew it for fifteen minutes only. If you make it stronger it may make you nauseous and, as it is particularly helpful for relieving the type of nausea associated with a bilious headache, that would be self-defeating! Adults should drink half a breakfast cup cold. Drunk warm after a meal as the French and Italians sometimes do, it will help digestion.

Like catnip, camomile is a particularly safe herb for children and babies and should be taken two teaspoons hourly, cold. It is a herb that mixes badly with allopathic medicines, so do not take it if you are still weaning yourself off these.

Catnip (Nepeta cataria)

My cat adores this plant and stalks me round the garden hoping I'll harvest some and so stir up its fragrance which makes her tremble with delight. A tea made with the pretty purple flowering tops is particularly good for strengthening the nervous system of children, and for this purpose is best mixed with equal parts of lemon balm and camomile. Cover the tea while infusing, so you don't lose any of the valuable volatile oils, and give three teaspoons hourly. I've given it in doses to fractious babies with digestive upsets with great success. A half cup sipped before bed will ensure a good night's sleep and allay nightmares. It can also be given as an enema where it will quickly act upon the nerves in the sacral plexus and, taken like this, is particularly effective in cases of hysteria when a child is having convulsions as the result of a screaming fit.

Hops (Humulus lupulus)

Strangely enough, hops were once believed actually to encourage the onset of melancholy. John Evelyn, the great diarist, admitted that hops preserved beer but added darkly, 'they repay the pleasure in tormenting diseases and a shorter life'! Those of us who enjoy the odd pint of bitter need not be alarmed, for it has since been discovered that the volatile oil in hops produces a soporific and sedative effect (as those of us who enjoy more than the odd few pints will know!). A standard infusion of hop leaves and stalks, mixed half and half with Earl Grey tea, is a reasonably palatable bedtime drink.

Hop pillows traditionally induce sleep but I've known patients suffer from stupor, dizziness and streaming eyes after trying one, so a woodruff pillow is preferable.

Lavender (Lavandula vera)

I cannot recommend lavender too highly as a headache cure. A drop of lavender oil rubbed into each temple will work almost magically, but do be very sparing about the amount you use. Measure your lavender oil in drops: in large doses it is a narcotic poison. If that warning has put you off using the oil, use lavender water instead. It can be splashed liberally on the forehead and temples and round the back of a tense, aching neck. Culpeper was obviously aware of the dire effect the liberal use of lavender oil might have when he wrote, 'the chymical oil drawn from Lavender, usually called Oil of Spike, is of so fierce and piercing a quality that it is cautiously to be used, some few drops being sufficient to be given with other things, either for inward or outward griefs'. Lavender oil works wonders added to warm bath water if you are suffering from nervous exhaustion. Add twenty drops to a warm bath, and soak, don't wash.

Lavender tea can also be used as a headache cure. Again be careful about the quantities of lavender you add to the water to make the tea, and never drink more than three cups a day. Add 10 g (⅓ oz) of the flowers to a litre (1¾ pt) of boiling water, infuse for five minutes only, strain and drink. The taste takes a little getting used to.

Lemon balm *(Melissa officinalis)*

This herb is good for insomnia, nervous headaches, and nervous depression because it eases anxiety. It also relieves the panicky feelings brought on by palpitations.

An infusion of lemon balm tea is best made from the fresh leaves, and tastes special if you add a squeeze of lemon juice and a curl of lemon peel. The dried leaves are a dusty, flavourless disappointment. For nervous disorders drink three cups of a standard infusion daily.

Linden *(Tilia europoea)*

Lime flowers need to be harvested in June and July – cut them well down on the stem so the whole bract is included. Dry them carefully in the shade, making sure they are unsullied by pollution (you'll often find them lining the streets, which is not the place to pick them) and use them up within six months. Ageing flowers can be poisonous. Taken as a standard infusion, a cup with each meal, and one more before bed, lime flowers are helpful for headaches which begin on the right side and then affect the left side and impair vision, for reducing high blood pressure which can often lead to dull, congested headaches, for soothing anxiety, and chronic insomnia. It is particularly effective in this last respect for old people and children and may be used in a bath, 1½ generous handfuls to 1 litre (1 ¾ pt) of water.

Marjoram, common *(Origanum majorana)*

This and the wild marjoram both have the same medicinal properties. Gerard recommended, 'the leaves boiled in water, and the decoction drunke, easeth such as are given to over-much sighing'. Certainly it is an excellent sedative and good for menstrual pain, nervous headaches and acid indigestion.

Use the flowering tips and be accurate about the dosage, as in strong doses it can be dangerous. Use an infusion of 40 g (1⅓ oz) to 1 litre (1¾ pt) water and take a cupful after each meal. A wine maceration of 50 g (1⅔ oz) to 1 litre (1¾ pt) of white wine left for ten days is very palatable. Take a sherry glassful after each meal. A hot fomentation wrapped round the abdomen will relieve the stressful pain of colic. If you can't grow it, the leaves, green dried, are almost as good.

Mistletoe *(Viscum album)*

This is an extraordinarily interesting plant. Its overall form is approximately spherical, unlike most other plants which are vertical. It is not influenced by gravity and has no real roots, attaching itself to the bark of trees with suckers and using their sap. Yet it is also capable of producing its own nourishment by using sunlight to convert carbon dioxide and water into sugar. It is green all year round and flowers in winter. All of this suggests a plant of a certain independence running counter to the normal rhythm of most plant life. No wonder the Druids revered it and harvested it from oak trees with golden knives and great ceremony. Nowadays you are far more likely to find it clinging to pear and apple trees, and indeed it is more effective when found growing on these trees than on any others. Modern research has shown it is valuable for the treatment of headaches and migraines due to high blood pressure because of its beneficial action on the vasomotor nervous system. It is also good for problems associated with arteriosclerosis, breathlessness, palpitations, angina, anxiety, and dizziness. But be warned. The berries are extremely poisonous, and overdoses of the leaves can result in numbness, slow paralysis and abdominal congestion, and may eventually lead to heart failure. So use only the green leaves and be very careful to pick out all berries. These are best harvested early in the autumn and dried in shade.

The active principles are partially destroyed by heat, so

prepare a cold infusion of 20 g (⅔ oz) of chopped leaves in ½ litre (1 pt) soaked for 12 hours. Strain and drink ¼ cupful before each meal. For external use to relieve the stressful pain of sciatica and neuralgia, use a cold compress of ½ handful of dried leaves to 1 litre (1¾ pt) water soaked for 24 hours.

Pulsatilla (Anemone pulsatilla)

A singularly lovely looking plant, this, with its violet flowers and silky leaves. Best used for very specific stress, for any undue sensitivity and weepiness, particularly in women going through the menopause badly, or those suffering from scanty menstruation, and for delicate children who like to be fussed over and can't sleep because they're afraid of the dark. It is also good for people who get into an emotional bind because they drive themselves too hard.

Use the whole plant collected shortly after flowering and make a wine maceration, 40 g (1 ⅓ oz) to 1 litre (1 ¾ pt) of wine, left to stand for 14 days. Ten drops in a little water, two or three times daily. If you have any left after a year, throw it away on your compost heap and start again because its medicinal action will begin to deteriorate.

Red clover (Trifolium pratense)

It has long been noted that cows seem particularly content when grazing in a clover field, hence the phrase 'living in clover'. I find clover tea, which is very pleasant tasting, excellent for stilling a carousel of anxiety exacerbated by exhaustion. Dr Fernie points out that it is rich in lime, silica and other mineral salts which would certainly help the tiredness nutritively. It is also useful for those who suffer from confusion or failing memory and often wake with headaches and a feeling of dread.

Collect the blossoms early in the morning when the dew is still on them. Infuse 20 g (⅔ oz) of the fresh flowers in a litre (1 ¾ pt) of boiling water for ten minutes. Strain and sweeten if possible with aromatic clover honey, which highlights the delicate taste of the flowers. Alternatively, use a few flowers shredded in a salad. Red clover tea made from dried flowers is also acceptable.

Rosemary (Rosmarinus officinalis)

In the very harsh winter we had a few years ago, I lost all my rosemary bushes in one fell swoop. Replacing them is proving a long, slow business as they grow so slowly. I'm particularly delighted with Jessops Upright and there are in fact many varieties of rosemary, but it is the green-leaved rosemary not the grey one that is used medicinally. It is one of the best-known headache cures and is good for vertigo, fainting, migraines and as a memory-specific. In the old days people breathed in the smoke from the burning branches for 'weyknesse of ye brayne', but there are more comfortable ways of ingesting it. Use 50 g (1⅔ oz) of the flowering tips to ½ litre (1 pt) of water and boil closely covered for two minutes. Leaving the lid on, let it stand for quarter of an hour. Drink ½ cupful twenty minutes before each meal. If you can't get the flowering tips, dried leaves will do.

Scullcap *(Scutellaria laterifolia)*

The beauty of scullcap is that it is very powerful but extremely safe. It bursts with minerals which contribute to its excellent action on the nervous system. I think it is one of the supreme remedies for nervous disorders and it works particularly well in combination with other appropriate herbs – vervain, hops, lady's slipper, wood betony.

It is good for high blood pressure, restlessness, an excitable twitch, headaches which spring from nervous disorders, hysteria, or for those who wake in the night suddenly, full of unnamed fears and premonitions of calamity. It is also useful for alcoholics and drug addicts trying to give up their particular poisons. It works very quickly if taken warm using fresh or dried leaves as an infusion – 50 g (1⅔ oz) to 1 litre (1¾ pt) water. Take ½ teacupful on waking and repeat the dose before bed.

Valerian *(Valeriana officinalis)*

The root smells obnoxiously of stale perspiration which is formed by the oxidation of the essential oil which, once it is exposed, turns into valerianic acid. Rats and cats love the smell.

It is the root that is mainly used to help relieve the sort of nervous exhaustion brought on by too much excitement which may result in palpitations, breathlessness, nervous contractions of the stomach, or migraine. It works particularly well combined with other herbs like camomile, vervain, woodruff, or lemon balm. If I administer it alone, I do so only in foot or hand baths.

Taken orally in isolation, it tends to depress the central nervous system and some patients react badly to this, becoming depressed and headachy. In overlarge doses, it will anyway cause severe headaches, mental agitation, heaviness and stupor. On the other hand, there are the odd few who find it unexpectedly stimulating, even in ordinary doses, and this is because their digestive enzymes are unable to transform valerian oil into the calming principles, valerianic acid.

Try to use the fresh root which is of greater medicinal value than the dried because it still has much of its own oil. As the roots are perennial, they should be allowed at least two years before being dug up. Having removed all the earth from the root by washing it thoroughly, slice up a level teaspoon as finely as you can and pour over half a litre (1 pt) of water which has been brought to boiling point but not actually allowed to boil. This subtle differentiation is very important as prolonged heat will dissipate the essential oils which are the principal healing ingredients. Cover and allow the tea to steep for 24 hours. Add an equal amount of another appropriate herb depending on the effect you want to achieve.

Vervain (Verbena officinalis)

Verbena officinalis is believed to be especially good for relieving the sort of prolonged mental stress which may show itself as constant severe headaches as well as tension in the neck and shoulders.

To make a vervain bath add 200 g (7 oz) of dried vervain leaves to 2 litres (3½ pt) of cold water. Bring to the boil then immediately remove from the stove. Leave to brew for fifteen minutes. Strain through a nylon sieve into your warm bath water. This makes a most refreshing bath, soothing away tension, especially round the neck and shoulders, so be sure to immerse yourself thoroughly in the water, putting a folded towel draped over the edge of the bath on which to rest your head. The towel will provide the extra grip you need to prevent yourself from slipping under the water altogether.

Vervain can also be drunk as tea. Make a decoction using 50 g (1¾ oz) to a litre (1¾ pt) of water. This can be drunk last thing at night to encourage sound sleep.

Alternatively, soak a flannel in the tea and apply it to the forehead and temples to soothe away headaches. A flannel and small towel immersed in the same tea, slightly wrung out and draped round the neck and shoulders, will also soothe away tension in this area, but do keep both yourself and the tea warm while you carry out this treatment, otherwise you will finish up with magnificently tension-free shoulders and severe rheumatism as the result of a cold soggy flannel being draped over your skin for a prolonged length of time. So keep this up for twenty minutes only, ensuring that the flannel, as it grows cool, is constantly replenished by a warm one dipped in hot infusion.

Woodruff (Asperula oderata)

This is a natural tranquilliser which soothes, calms and relaxes, and is especially good for people suffering from extreme nervous tension which prevents them sleeping. The leaves only exude their inimitable odour, redolent of new-mown hay and honey with a hint of vanilla, once they are dry, so this fragrant herb can be used to stuff pillows. Alternatively, keep muslin sachets of woodruff permanently in your linen cupboard to scent all your sheets. The fragrance will last even when the sheets have been on the bed for two or three days. I have always found woodruff a much more satisfactory sleep-inducing herb than hops. Restless toddlers particularly appreciate a thin pillow stuffed with dried woodruff and laid over the top of their own pillows. If the cover of the case is strong, it isn't prickly to lie on.

Combinations of herbs for specific problems

If your problem is more complex than insomnia or a headache you may find certain combinations of herbs are necessary.

Drug addiction

Hoffman LaRoche sell about 300 million Valium and Librium tranquillisers a year in the UK alone. That's about ten for every adult in the country, but as this number is obviously not proportionate, there must be a lot of long-term addicts around. Indeed, the World Health Organisation says there are two million long-term depressed people in Britain. If you're on tranquillisers or artificial stimulants, *wean yourself off them gently*. Hauling yourself straight off a ten-year Valium dependency is asking for trouble. I cannot emphasise this strongly enough. It is possible to become addicted to tranquillisers in a few short months. Reversing the process takes time and persistence and must be done slowly.

As you reduce your dosage, support your nervous system with a regular routine, a good diet, plenty of exercise, and loving friends with whom you enjoy a confiding relationship. Then incorporate a really good tranquilliser into your diet. It should not be poisonous, addictive, suppressive, produce side-effects, dull the senses or stupefy the brain. It should soothe, nourish, and rebuild the nervous system. Certain herbs do all of these things and more.

All addictive drugs need to be withdrawn gradually, and this particularly applies to the common tranquillisers. Use the same system of treatment as for alcoholism, but do not begin your two-week fast until you have at least halved the dosage of drugs by using the formulation for alcoholism coupled with a good mucusless diet, meaning no processed or refined products whatsoever, no dairy products, salt, sugar, red meat, tea, coffee or chocolate, all of which are addictive in themselves or clog up the system and impede the cleansing process.

Depression formula

    3 parts lemon balm (*Melissa officinalis*)
    1 part passion flower (*Passiflora incarnata*)
    2 parts cornsilk (*Zea mays*)
    1 part peppermint (*Mintha piperita*)
    1 part lady's slipper (*Cypripedium pubescens*)
    1 part vervain (*Verbena officinalis*)

Infuse and drink ¾ cups daily between meals. Skin brush twice daily and go barefoot walking. This tea will soothe and rebuild the nervous system, assist the kidneys and the skin to flush toxins out of the body and it is rich in minerals, particularly calcium which will repair frayed nerves.

Exhaustion formula

    4 parts alfalfa (*Medicago sativa*)
    1 part sage (*Salvia officinalis*)
    1 part solomon's seal (*Polygonatum multiflorum*)
    1 part Irish moss (*Chondrus crispus*)
    1 part bayberry (*Myrica cerifera*)

1 part rosemary (*Rosmarinus officinalis*)

Make a decoction using 1 oz to 1 pt. Add 1 tbsp black strap molasses and 1 tbsp glycerine. Bottle and store in fridge. Take 1 tbsp 4 or 5 times daily. Ensure your nutrition is particularly good and that you're getting lots of iron, calcium and magnesium in particular.

This formulation is abundant in vitamins and minerals which will help to combat any weakness or deficiencies in the body, it will assist a sluggish liver and get the circulation working properly, encouraging blood into the brain. It will also ensure the digestive tract is assimilating food appropriately.

Failing memory formula

1 part scullcap (*Scutellaria spp*)
3 parts gota kola (*Centella asiatica*)
1 part lady's slipper (*Cypripedium pubescens*)
2 parts rosemary (*Rosmarinus officinalis*)
1 part wood betony (*Betonica officinalis*)
1 part ginger (*Zingiber officinale*)

Take two size '00' capsules with each meal. Ensure your glandular system is in peak condition (see page 151). Plenty of skin brushing and scalp massage and, twice daily, slant board exercises (see page 288). The rosemary and gota kola are particularly effective for loss of memory while ginger is stimulating. The remaining herbs will calm and assist the nervous system.

Smoking

There's no need to offer a litany of all the terrible things that happen to you as a result of this bad habit. The crux of the matter is, how can one give up? The most effective way to do so is to go on a fruit juice fast for two weeks under the supervision of a person experienced in these matters, and to have some calamus root standing by. If you feel desperately in need of a lungful of tobacco smoke, chew a little of the root. You'll find if you try to smoke afterwards the taste of tobacco will make you feel sick. The following formula will also help you give up smoking if juice-fasting is impossible for you:

1 part oatstraw (*Avena sativa*)
1 part lobelia (*Lobelia inflata*)
2 parts lemon balm (*Melissa officinalis*)
1 part liquorice (*Glycyrrhiza glabra*)

Take one size '00' capsule every three hours until the worst of the craving is gone, and then reduce to one size '0' capsules three times daily **with** meals. Don't skip meals. Once you feel you are well in control of yourself, stop taking the herbs.

This formulation will help expel some of the accumulated nicotine through the skin and via the kidneys, it is rich in soothing calcium and other minerals which will work to rebuild the nervous system, and it will relieve lung congestion. The lobelia in it is particularly helpful for breaking the smoking habit.

Alcoholism

Surprising though it may sound, alcoholism may well be the result of nutritional deficiencies. In other words, these deficiencies don't follow as the result of heavy alcohol intake but predispose a person to alcoholism. Early warning signs include hypoglycaemia, adrenal exhaustion and chronic fatigue, where alcohol is used to kick-start the body.

The easiest way to break the alcohol habit is to fast for a fortnight and then go onto a supremely nutritious diet. Use protein snacks like nuts or yoghurt to overcome the craving for a lift. Get plenty of rest and take as much exercise as you can comfortably manage, preferably out of doors. Massage also helps. So if you can find a good masseur, take full advantage. Concentrate on plenty of skin brushing. The following formulation will help with the DTs or withdrawal symptoms, and is also helpful for modifying drug withdrawal symptoms while strengthening and helping to rebuild the nervous system. Equal parts of:

lady's slipper (*Cypripedium pubescens*)
lemon balm (*Melissa officinalis*)
scullcap (*Scutellaria spp*)
wood betony (*Betonica officinalis*)
vervain (*Verbena officinalis*)

Make a decoction. Take half a cup hourly if the withdrawal symptoms are bad. Otherwise one cup on rising and one before bed.

CHAPTER 7

Children

How to administer herbs to a baby

Babies react very positively to herbal medicine and a little goes a long way. It isn't just because they're much smaller than adults and therefore need proportionately smaller doses, but because their systems are less contaminated by the self-indulgent rubbish we've tended to throw into ours over the years, so that they are far more receptive to the gentle action of herbs. Because of their sensitivity it is best to administer herbs externally as far as possible, in the form of baths, poultices, fomentations and massage. Otherwise herbs can be given in diluted infusions as teas, or if the baby's being breastfed, indirectly through the mother's milk by the mother taking the necessary herbs.

Herbal baths for babies

I've never met a baby who didn't love the water. Indeed my god-daughter creates a loud fuss when, to her mind, she's hauled out of the bath too soon. Water should be tepid at about blood heat, and you can add cooled decoctions of the following herbs to the bath: about half the quantity of the water should be made up of the strained decoction.

Camomile (Matricaria chamomilla) for digestive upsets, restlessness, and gastric pains.

Marigold (Calendula officinalis) for skin rashes and itching.

181

Lemon balm (Melissa officinalis) or *lime flowers (Tilia europoea)* to soothe and calm a fractious baby.

Lady's mantle (Alchemilla vulgaris) if the skin is flabby and in poor condition, or if there is a tendency to hernias.

Wild thyme (Thymus serpyllum) to correct a pulmonary weakness or if the baby catches cold easily.

Plantain (Plantago lanceolata) if you suspect the child has a weak bladder, though this will not be possible to confirm until toilet training is completed.

Golden rod (Solidago virgaurea) if you think the baby has caught a chill over the kidneys.

Rose (Roseaceae) or *lavender (Lavandula vera)* are both soothing and strengthening.

Do not lay the baby so far back that the ears are at risk of getting obstructed with tiny remnants of floating herbs, as with camomile or lime flowers, which are very difficult to strain completely. Hold the baby by the right hand so that the left arm is across the chest and not dangling down over the stomach. Make sure the head is supported. Use a very mild soap only if you absolutely have to, but it is better to wash just with the herbal water or a lightly scented bag of wet oatmeal. After washing, bounce the palms of the baby's hands and soles of the feet up and down gently with your own palms to stimulate the nerve endings there, which will in turn gently stimulate the rest of the body. Dry gently with a soft towel, first lying the baby on the tummy and then on the back, and don't feel inhibited about singing gently to her or even crooning if you're not blessed with a great voice.

Don't use talcum powder because it simply absorbs the urine and encourages the growth of bacteria, and the child may inhale too much of it which could be dangerous. Oiling is far preferable and prevents soreness much more effectively. Use St John's wort or rose oil with almond or olive oil added (10 drops of the essential oil to a teaspoon of the other, and 2 or 3 drops of cider vinegar), and massage well into the bottom and legs. Once the baby is a month old, you can enjoy the pleasure of massaging with this oil all over. Pay special attention to the child's eyes and nose, and keep them clean and lightly lubricated. Put a tiny dab of rosewater, mixed half and half with almond oil, over the baby's eyelids, being careful not to let it run into the eyes, and add a small dab to each nostril. If eyes get gummy and sore, bathe in an infusion of cornflowers or marshmallow which has been carefully freshly made with purified water. Don't use an eye bath. Wipe the lids with clean, soaked gauze.

If the weather is clement, it's a good idea to do this massage outside, so the baby can enjoy an air and sun bath. Point the feet towards the sun, and if it is hot or bright, protect both your own and the baby's head with an umbrella.

Caution

Babies are super-sensitive to any medication, and any herbs administered should be very weak so that their delicate constitutions are not upset. If an infusion is to be given in a feeding bottle or disguised in juice, prepare it by adding ⅛th of a level teaspoonful of herb to one cup of water.

Babies' ailments (in alphabetical order)

Colic

Give catnip and fennel infusion, ⅛th of a teaspoon of the two herbs mixed to 1 cup of water, administering a teaspoon every five minutes until the worst of the pain is over. Then space the dose to one teaspoon every half hour until the colic subsides. Meanwhile keep the baby's stomach warm and, if you can, give an enema of 2 oz in all of a well-strained, ordinary strength, lukewarm catnip infusion. That is, make up an infusion using 1 oz of the herb to 1 pt of water, brew as usual and then strain and measure out 2 fl oz.

Look to improving your own diet. One theory suggests that colic rarely occurs in a baby unless the mother has been on such an inadequate diet during pregnancy that her baby's adrenal glands are exhausted. So take the adrenal formulation (see page 256) and drink lots of peppermint tea. Mothers should follow the dietary advice in Chapter 1 and should certainly cut out dairy products. Calcium is richly abundant from other sources (see page 96).

Constipation

Equal parts of: ˙

> slippery elm (*Ulmus fulva*)
> fennel (*Foeniculum vulgare*)
> turkey rhubarb (*Rheum palmatum*)
> liquorice (*Glycyrrhiza glabra*)

Mix with equal quantities of carob powder. Feed ¼ teaspoonful mixed to a thin paste in a little water once or twice daily. If the baby is not eating at all, take the lower bowel tonic yourself and breastfeed the baby. This is very effective.

Cradle cap

If the child is no longer breastfeeding, check there are no dairy products in the diet. Give 4 tsps of a standard infusion of heartsease (*Viola tricolor*) with every feed and ensure there is plenty of calcium in the diet, if necessary adding the calcium formula sprinkled into oat or millet cereals (see page 258).

If the baby is still at the breast, ensure you drink 1 pint of almond milk daily (soak 1 oz (28 g) of freshly-grated almonds in 1 pt (½ litre) of water for 24 hours and drink the juice). Add the almond sludge to cereals or soups. Ensure your intake of magnesium and B_6 are adequate. Crush 100 mg B_6 to a fine powder and add to 1 tbsp almond oil. Rub gently over the yellow crusty scabs. Alternatively, wash the head with a tepid standard infusion of meadow-sweet flowers.

Diarrhoea

Feed slippery elm gruel sweetened with a touch of honey with a tiny pinch of ginger or cinnamon added.

Digestive upsets

Make a tea of dill or anise seed, using ⅛th tsp of the herbs to 1 cup of water and preparing it as a decoction. Add a tiny pinch of ginger or cinnamon. Give as much of this as the baby will comfortably drink.

Nutritional problems

Start as you mean to go on by feeding the baby only the best possible food. My god-daughter loves avocados or bananas mashed into millet, and took to freshly juiced fruit and vegetables with alacrity. Many babies enjoy nut-milks and most like herbal teas. Once the child can chew, forty per cent of the diet should be raw. Before this you might consider chewing the food for your baby, and when it is finely pulped, passing it over in a spoon. In this way you've begun the first stage of digestion for the baby and no, it is not at all unhygienic and disgusting! In my own childhood I saw African women doing this for their babies, only they used their fingers on which to spit out the food and pass it on, and their babies thrived.

Many babies don't take well to citrus fruits and berries, so try these out cautiously at first and watch for reactions. Most love apple purée. Vegetables, including baked mashed potatoes scooped out of their skins, are also acceptable, but it is advisable to cook those high in oxalic acid (spinach, broccoli, cauliflower, kale and cabbage) in a little goat's milk to neutralise it.

Be very cautious with honey while the child is less than a year old. In a few babies it can cause 'honey botulism', a misnomer really, as true botulism is caused by rotting food. Some babies experience severe gastric upset with raw honey, and of course anything which is very sweet can be addictive. So herbal teas should be served plain or with only a touch of honey.

An older child's diet should consist of plenty of fruit and vegetables, cereals, nuts and sprouted seeds with honey, black strap molasses and maple syrup for sweetness. Don't deny them sweets and ice lollies, just be imaginative about how you make them, the former with dried fruit, honey, nuts and carob, and the latter with fresh juice frozen in moulds.

Be careful about comforting an ill, emotional or upset child with food, otherwise they may learn the bad habits of 'comfort' eating. If the child is upset, cuddles and talking, or a brisk walk outside is a better way of dissipating furious pent-up energy.

Teething

Rubbing the gums with a little honey and a pinch of salt may take away some of the pain, but generally you'll find you'll need stronger measures. Try letting the child chew on a piece of arrowroot, liquorice or marshmallow root. Not too much liquorice or the bowels will get very loose. If the pain is very bad, rub two or three drops of essential oil of camomile into the gums, having just mixed it with honey as the taste is very powerful.

Diarrhoea while teething

Mix equal parts of the following seeds:

> dill (*Pencedanum graveolens*)
> anise (*Pimpinella anisum*)
> caraway (*Carum carvi*)
> fennel (*Foeniculium vulgare*)

Pound as finely as possible in a pestle and mortar. Add enough slippery elm gruel to mix to a poultice consistency and spread over the stomach. Give no other food or drinks until the worst of the diarrhoea has subsided, except weak yarrow tea (½ oz/16 g to 1 pt/½ litre water). 4 teaspoons every 20 minutes. If the diarrhoea simply won't pass off properly, feed the child slippery elm made into a thin gruel with yarrow tea.

Thrush

This is usually much more common among the bottle-fed babies, doubly so if the mother had thrush during pregnancy. So to ensure you are free of this prior to conception, strengthen the reproductive organs and faithfully adhere to a course of vaginal boluses and douching (see Chapter 11).

Bottle-fed babies need to be fed diluted live yoghurt and rejuvelac (see page 17). Their mouths need to be rinsed out with a decoction of white oak bark regularly. Breastfed babies need to be fed vitamins through the mother's milk, and the same procedure followed with white oak bark. Mother should take 6 g sustained-release vitamin C daily, 1 B complex and 100 mg niaciniamode. Under no circumstances should a woman prone to thrush take oral antibiotics which wipe out the friendly bacteria in the lower colon altogether, leaving an ideal breeding ground for *Candida albicans* and *Monilia albicans*. If you need an antibiotic, see page 276, or take the following formulation, which is Dr Vogel's.

Equal parts of:

butterburr (*Petasites hybridus*)
nasturtium (*Tropaeolum majus*)
horseradish (*Cochlearia armoracia*)
watercress (*Nasturtium officinalis*)
garden cress (*Lepidium sativum*)

Make into a standard tincture (see page 128) and take 1 teaspoon (5 ml) three times a day before meals.

Vomiting

If it is projectile, that is, shoots across the room, see your doctor immediately because it may be pyloric stenosis – that is, a narrowing of the opening into the stomach. If the baby is vomiting through sheer greed by gulping down breast milk too quickly, wash out the mouth with a standard infusion of dill, and feed sips of this with a pinch of cloves added.

How to administer herbs to children

Toddlers and children can be given herbs in proportionately tailored doses in the same way as adults will take them, though many will prefer their tinctures, which tend to taste bitter, disguised in fruit juice and their herb powders hidden in electuaries. Perhaps I've just been exceptionally lucky with the children I've treated, but I've found most of them will willingly take the herbal medicine if the reason why they're having to take it is explained to them in a way in which they can understand. The worst obstacles to getting children to take herbs are, in my experience at least, frightened or over-indulgent mothers. So administer the herbal medicine calmly to the child and don't make a fuss. Praise the child for accepting the herb easily.

Correct dosage for children

To determine this divide the child's next birthday by 24. So a dose for a three-year-old would be: $4/24 = 1/6$th of the adult dose.

For example, if a formulation calls for 1 cup of a herbal tea three times daily for an adult, this would mean $1/6$th of a cup of herbal tea for a three-year-old three times daily. If it calls for 60 drops of tincture three times daily, the amount for a three-year-old would be 10 drops. If it calls for 2 size '00' capsules 3 times daily for an adult, a three-year-old would take 1 size '00' capsule once during the course of the day. If the '00' size was too large to swallow (as is likely to be the case with a three-year-old) give 2 size '0' capsules in the course of the day instead, one in the morning and one at night.

Childhood ailments (in alphabetical order)

Anaemia

> 3 parts yellow dock (*Rumex crispus*)
> 1 part burdock (*Arctium lappa*)
> 1 part comfrey (*Symphytum officinale*)
> 1 part nettles (*Urtica urens*)

Mix and make a standard decoction. Sweeten, as most children won't take it unadulterated, and give two tablespoons after every meal. Ensure the child eats plenty of iron-rich foods like beetroot, red grapes and juices, raisins, watercress and seeds with green sprouts. Add freshly pressed nettle juice to soups in the spring, or serve the young tops cooked like spinach. Encourage lots of fresh air and exercise.

Asthma

Absolutely no refined or starchy foods, eggs or dairy products. Lots of iodine-rich foods, garlic and onions; meals should be little and often, as many asthmatics are also hypoglycaemic.

> 1 part Irish moss (*Chondrus crispus*)
> 1 part Iceland moss (*Cetraria islandica*)
> 1 part horehound (*Marrubium vulgare*)
> 1 part thyme (*Thymus vulgaris*)
> 1 part red clover (*Trifolium pratense*)
> 1 part liquorice (*Glycyrrhiza glabra*)
> ¼ part cayenne (*Capsicum annum*)

Make a standard decoction. Strain, pressing down well as the moss tends to retain a lot of liquid. Reduce by one-third and add a tablespoon of black strap molasses and a teaspoon of glycerine. Cool. Bottle. A teaspoon every hour until relief is obtained, or one teaspoon four times a day as a prophylactic. If a bad attack comes directly after a meal, make the child vomit by giving a cup of peppermint tea followed by a teaspoon of lobelia tincture. If the child is in pain, give a level teaspoon of half-pounded linseed mixed with honey, and rub the chest with linseed oil (not the sort used to season cricket bats, but the unadulterated linseed you can get from a chemist).

About a quarter of all young asthmatics are believed to have a deep-seated emotional insecurity and an intense need for parental love and protection. If you suspect your child falls into this category, try and get it sorted out. Also be alert for sources of possible allergies – house mites which hide in blankets, mattresses and carpets, cats and other animal dust and feathers.

Deep breathing exercises are helpful and, once learned, a useful way to help control the panicky feeling induced by an attack. A daily herbal steam bath of wormwood, vervain and rosemary in equal parts is also beneficial.

Bedwetting

Do not give the child anything after seven o'clock. If she is thirsty, offer a really juicy piece of fruit instead. There must be absolutely no salt in the diet. Massage the kidneys daily with warm almond oil and encourage her to sleep on her side, not on her back. Give three cups of equal parts of parsley and corn tassle tea daily. This is a particularly safe remedy for children because it won't irritate tender tummies or the urinary tract, so making the problem worse. Foot baths of the tassles from corn on the cob also help. There really isn't any need to worry about bedwetting unless it is persistent beyond the age of six or seven.

Chickenpox

Treat as for fever and measles (see page 195). Cider vinegar rub-downs will help a little with the unbearable itching as an alternative to golden seal.

Colds and Influenza

Get the child to drink as much as she can of equal parts of elderflower, yarrow and peppermint tea. Give a gram of vitamin C hourly (the chewable sort goes down better with children). These are available from health food shops and are marked 'chewable' on the label. This is slightly laxative, so you need not worry about clearing the bowel. If the child is really poorly and complains of aching bones, it is likely she has the 'flu. Put her to bed and give her a standard infusion of boneset (*Eupatorium perfoliatum*) tea, half a cup at a time until she's sweating well. Persist even if she vomits and don't be alarmed or feel horrid having to do this; vomiting is just the body's way of clearing itself. Let her rest once she's sweating, and resume treatment if she stops until she's well. When not drinking boneset, let her drink raspberry tea instead. Sponge the body down every few hours with an infusion of thyme and lime flowers in equal parts.

Constipation
Make sure the child is getting plenty of raw food every day and drinking lots of purified water, and administer the stomach massage daily using olive oil and turning the routine into a pleasant game. Give the lower bowel tonic on page 143 in appropriate doses disguised in an electuary.

Coughs
If in any doubt at all about the underlying cause, consult a medical herbalist. If the cough is the result of a cold or a chill, make a standard infusion of:

> 2 parts hyssop (*Hyssopus officinalis*)
> 2 parts marshmallow (*Althaea officinalis*)
> 2 parts coltsfoot(*Tussilago farfara*)
> 2 parts horehound (*Marrubium vulgare*)
> 1 part peppermint (*Mintha piperita*)
> 1 part liquorice (*Glycyrrhiza glabra*)

Sweeten well with lots of honey. Give the child one tablespoon every hour, if the child is over ten, and reduce the dose proportionally for younger children.

If the cough is a racking one and keeps everyone, including the poor child, awake at night, try a syrup of:

> 3 parts wild cherry bark (*Prunus serotina*)
> 1 part coltsfoot (*Tussilago farfara*)
> 1 part camomile (*Matricaria chamomilla*)
> 1 part plantain (*Plantago spp*)
> 1 part lobelia (*Lobelia inflata*)

Give one teaspoon every fifteen minutes for children over ten and reduce the dose proportionately for younger children. Encourage the child to drink plenty of fresh blackcurrant juice.

Diarrhoea

See page 184 in the section on babies and adjust the dose according to the age of the child, or simply feed the child as much gruel as she'll take. There's no danger in overdosing.

Earache

Ears are very delicate, sensitive, complex organs and can easily be permanently damaged by neglect or inappropriate treatment. If you're in any doubt about the cause of the earache, consult your doctor. This is particularly important in the case of babies, who can't tell you what is wrong but can only scratch at their ears or pull them or, more likely, yell. If the earache is the result of a chill, apply a raw grated onion poultice over the back and side of the neck, securing with a cotton bandage. Drop a few drops of mullein oil into both ears, even if the earache is only in one ear, and plug with cotton wool. Keep the head, neck and ears warm at all times. Keep the child on a fruit diet for a few days.

If the child is particularly prone to earaches, consider a three-month nightly course of mullein and lobelia poultices (see page 131) to get it cleared up once and for all, and during this time include lots of garlic in a diet which should consist only of fruits, vegetables, nuts, grains and sprouted seeds, eighty per cent of these raw. Also give mullein and lobelia in tea form and work on cleansing the lymphatic system (see page 154).

Eczema

The causes of eczema are many and varied, and it is important to consider the conditions of the lymph and blood and to check that the bowels, liver and kidneys are working properly. Many children who have eczema are often, at least in my experience, extremely sensitive to all dairy products, wheat and citrus fruits, so it is best to get them to follow a diet as for earache and to offer grain only in sprouted or low-heated form, not as bread. Ensure there is plenty of calcium in the diet, calcium-rich herbs and sweets made from sesame seeds, which seem to go down particularly well with children. If the child can't chew properly yet, substitute tahini. Wash only with oatmeal or rice bran bags, and rub the area externally with essential oil of roses mixed with sesame oil or chickweed ointment. Give a good blood-purifying tea such as red clover blossom, also three cups of heartsease (*Viola tricolor*) tea daily. Herbs like artichoke leaves, chickweed, comfrey, lime flowers, plantain, walnut leaves, blackberry or strawberry leaves added to the water also help.

If the itching gets unbearable, apply a poultice of yoghurt, or better still, whey, in which you have macerated finely grated carrot and horseradish root for an hour. Strain out the vegetable matter before applying. In an emergency, dab on diluted, freshly squeezed lemon juice. Calendula cream made from marigolds, which can be bought ready prepared, is sometimes helpful.

Fevers

These are a God-given way of burning up and expelling all sorts of poisons which have accumulated in the body and, contrary to current medical dogma, **should not be suppressed**. However, nature will need a little help with enemas and sweat-inducing teas sometimes. If fevers are suppressed, the purifying processes will be nipped in the bud, laying up trouble for the future. Work with the fever, not against it, but do so intelligently. A high temperature must not be allowed to get out of control. Sponge down the skin with a mixture of three-quarters cool water and one-quarter of apple cider vinegar.

Check that the bowels are open and working freely. If not, administer an enema of rue, wormwood, horsetail, rosemary or yarrow. If the child raises the roof and refuses the enema, administer equal quantities of turkey rhubarb and fennel, finely powdered and hidden in an electuary in the appropriate dose.

Give the child plenty of warm honey and lemon, or cider vinegar drinks. If the child can stand it, crush a clove of garlic into the drink and add a pinch of ginger. Do not feed the child at all or offer any cold drinks. If the child has a high temperature and is not sweating, use yarrow and elderflower tea to induce a sweat and bring the temperature down. Apply warm ginger fomentations over the kidneys if necessary (see page 149). All fabrics in the bed and next to the skin should be natural.

If the problem is heavy catarrh on the chest, apply thyme fomentations over the lungs (for instructions on how to make up a fomentation see page 132), and garlic paste on the soles of the feet. Crush two big cloves of garlic into a dessertspoon of vaseline and spread the paste over the soles of the feet only, not over the entire foot. Wrap the feet in cotton bandages to hold the garlic in place, and then put on a pair of white cotton or woollen socks. Leave on all night, though of course the thyme fomentations are to be removed once cool.

The next morning sponge the skin down with a half-and-half mixture of cider vinegar and lavender infusion. Into clean nightwear and back to bed. Offer plenty of freshly pressed, not chilled fruit and vegetable juices. When the child's appetite comes back, offer soupy grains or steamed fruit, though not in the same meal, and a week's course of rejuvelac. Once the child will swallow, offer an antibiotic tailoring the dose according to age; (see page 187) three times a day, and keep up the whole course for two weeks (see page 276). While the fever is present, keep the room coolish and shaded to protect the child's eyes. Ensure plenty of bed-rest for a few days after a fever. (Easier said than done, as any child who has gone through a fever well will be raring to go again very soon afterwards.)

When to use enemas for children

The fact that many children don't take easily to enemas should not deter you from giving them if they are necessary. They can be invaluable for the treatment of certain illnesses like fevers, when the colon needs to be cleared of faeces as quickly as possible to accelerate the healing process. If a child adamantly refuses an enema, then give the lower bowel tonic instead (see page 143), but this is less preferable as it takes much longer to work. It helps to explain to the child that an enema is necessary to clean out all waste from the colon so that they can get better much more quickly.

Caution

Do not administer enemas to children under five yourself. Seek the advice and the practical help of a professional person experienced in these matters.

How to give an enema to a child

Lie the child on her left-hand side with knees bent. Expel all the air out of the kit if using a bulb, or make sure the herb tea is flowing freely if using a kit. Grease the nozzle with a little vaseline, and gently insert it into the anus with a push and a quick sideways twist. Young children should not take in more than ¼ pt (⅛ litre), and the liquid should always be at body temperature. Children over ten can take ¾ pint. Don't ask the child to try and retain the enema. Just sit her on a potty or the toilet and let it go. If it looks as if the child can retain the enema for a short while, gently roll her over and, with warm olive oil, massage the colon backwards rhythmically to encourage the enema to penetrate right down to the bottom of the ascending colon. Then encourage the child to expel it.

German measles
Dab the skin with a strong infusion (2 oz to 1 pt) of yarrow. Apply tincture of golden seal or tincture of marigold locally on spots which are uncomfortably itchy. Give tincture of black colosh in fruit juice every six hours, so work out your child's dose accurately and give appropriately.

Hiccups
This tends to be a problem in children only when they eat food which ferments in the stomach and causes gas, or if they're full of phlegm. Ensure fruit and juices are not taken with any meals, though they may be eaten or drunk separately an hour or more after a meal. See the section of food combinations on page 34. Meals should be eaten in a quiet calm atmosphere at a leisurely pace.

You will know the one about drinking cold water out of the wrong side of a glass. It often works. If it doesn't, try giving equal parts of fennel or anise or dill and roses boiled as a decoction, a teaspoon at a time. Especially suitable for babies. Freshly grated coconut, if you have it to hand, mixed with an equal part of solid honey is good for toddlers. Make sure it is chewed well.

Insomnia
If this is because the baby is constantly crying, first check all the obvious possibilities – heat, cold, hunger, thirst, digestive or urinary difficulties, safety pins stuck in flesh, uncomfortable wet nappies, boredom, and remedy them accordingly. If none of this applies, work your way through a series of the gentlest solutions – baths in camomile, lemon balm or lime flowers after a very light supper. A mattress stuffed with plenty of freshly picked woodruff helps or, if the child is not yet potty-trained, a thin

flattish pillow of the same. Bedrooms should be kept warm, but there must be room for fresh air to circulate freely. A rocking cradle; a night light; cups of the gentler sleep-inducing teas with supper – lemon balm, catnip, vervain, camomile, lime flowers, woodruff.

If none of these measures are proving effective, graduate to a couple of drops of tincture of lobelia added to these teas, or two drops of essential oil of camomile in a little brown sugar. Or administer the following tea in appropriate doses (see page 187).

> 1 part camomile (*Matricaria chamomilla*)
> 1 part scullcap (*Scultaria spp*)
> 1 part vervain (*Verbena officinalis*)
> 1 part peppermint (*Mintha piperita*)
> 2 parts woodruff (*Asperula oderata*)

You'll probably need a stronger version of this if the disruption has been going on for some time (see page 126).

Measles

Treat as for fever, but if the child is slow in breaking out, apply hot fomentations of thyme to the skin to draw out the rash. Instead of yarrow and elderflower tea, use yarrow, borage and catnip in equal parts freely. If the eyes are sore, bathe with equal parts of cornflower and eyebright and shade the room. If the itching is unbearable, dab on tincture of golden seal locally. It will stain the skin, but not permanently.

Mumps

Treat as for fever and apply a fomentation over the swelling of three parts of mullein leaves to one part of lobelia. This is Dr Christopher's formulation, and I've used it very successfully on swollen glands. Offer horsetail tea. If mullein and lobelia is not available, soak a cloth in St John's wort infusion and apply it warm as a fomentation, changing frequently.

Nits

Massage the scalp with essential oil of thyme diluted with a little alcohol. The correct proportion is ten drops to one teaspoon of vodka. Leave this mixture on overnight, protecting the pillow with a towel and wrapping up the child's head in a scarf, and wash out the next morning. Comb the hair with a specially fine comb designed to take out eggs from the hair. Repeat this treatment until the scalp is clear.

It is often the cleanest scalp and hair that succumbs to head lice, so don't be embarrassed about this.

Styes

Check the bowels are working properly. Bathe the eyes with equal parts of a decoction of eyebright, burdock and sarsaparilla, and give the child this mixture internally according to age. If the stye is unbearably itchy, rub it with a piece of raw potato or, if you can get it, the clean cut edge of a piece of fresh marshmallow root.

Toothache

If the face is swollen, apply warm poultices of onion, catnip, or camomile to the puffy areas and over the back of the neck. Put a drop of essential oil of cloves or marjoram onto the tooth and massage another in the surrounding gum, or get the child to chew on a whole clove or a few yarrow leaves, or some prickly ash bark, using the teeth that are causing the pain. A tablet of betain hydrochloride crushed and spread over the tooth also affords remarkable relief.

If the glands are swollen, apply a warm poultice of mullein over them and across the back of the neck, and give frequent sips of mullein tea.

As an emergency measure you can plug any cavity with a small sliver of fresh horseradish root or garlic until you can get the child to a dentist, although when I told my own dentist about that he observed ruefully that it might be kinder to the dentist to use a sugar-free chewing gum instead.

Abscesses can be cleared by:

2 parts echinacea (*Echinacea angustifolia*)
1 part burdock (*Arctium lappa*)
1 part yellow dock (*Rumex crispus*)
1 part liquorice (*Glycyrrhiza glabra*)
½ part cloves (*Eugenia aromatisa*)

Children under ten – one size 2 capsule every hour. Double the dose for those over ten. Children under five – ten drops of the tincture every hour. This will cleanse the blood and lymph system and is mildly antiseptic.

All children should have lots of natural calcium (see page 95) daily, as should pregnant mums. It pays priceless dividends.

Travel sickness

Give the child a cup of freshly grated ginger-root tea and honey before a journey, and feed home-made ginger biscuits while travelling. Lots of fresh air is also helpful, and distracting games which involve the brain and voice but not the eyes. Reading while travelling is fatal except in a large aircraft.

Correct toothbrushing

Begin as you mean to go on and teach the child the right way to brush teeth. Use a soft brush with rounded bristles spread with a little herbal toothpaste. The brush should be held at an angle of 45° to the teeth which should be *gently* scrubbed following this angle. The mouth can be rinsed with infusions of verbena, lavender or violet or with a few drops of tincture of myrrh in water. Once the child is old enough to use dental floss after the second teeth have come through, it should be used daily, again gently, to dislodge any plaque. This should be done before any brushing and should be followed by a good gum massage using the fingertip in small, rotary circles. A few nuts are a good way of ending a meal because they leave the mouth in a non-acidic condition, which is less likely to help corrosion than the acid left in the mouth by munching apples, carrots or celery.

If there's no toothpaste to be had, use sage leaves freshly picked and rubbed over the teeth.

Warts

The best thing I know of to cure warts is the fresh yellow juice of greater celandine (*Chelidonium majus*). I'm afraid the dried plant won't do. Paint the skin surrounding the warts with vaseline, then dab on the fresh juice over the warts and cover with a plaster or a bandage. Change the dressing at least twice daily and renew the juice. In a week or so the wart should soften and eventually disappear. Don't let children taste the juice. It is extremely poisonous.

Other remedies which I haven't used, but which are said to be effective, are the juice from the stalks of fig leaves, the inner side of pineapple peel, the sap from marigold leaves, and the juice from bluebell flowers.

Whooping cough

This sounds like no other cough, so when you hear the child barking sharply and then breathing in deeply with a sort of sonorous, whooping sound, act on it quickly. Treat as for fever and offer equal parts of cayenne and garlic hidden in honey, small frequent nibbles to clear the throat. Apply poultices of onion and horseradish equally mixed over the chest, and remove as soon as the skin is red. Two drops of tincture of lobelia in a tablespoon of thyme tea every half hour will help to get the phlegm up. Alternatively, Michael Tierra, a superb American herbalist, suggests equal parts of elecampagne, black cohosh and wild cherry bark administered in tincture form. Take five drops six times daily with a cup of coltsfoot tea for a ten-year-old. Be meticulous about the dosage. Too large a dose and the child may suffer from dizziness and vomiting.

Worms

Worms are surprisingly common in children, though, as with head lice, most fastidious mothers would be hard-pressed to acknowledge this, partly because children often don't show any obvious symptoms. The most common way of picking up worms is from other children, but they can also be picked up from insufficiently cooked meat or fish, from dogs licking hands or faces, from manure, and a diet heavy in processed starchy food; sugar and fat will only encourage them.

Symptoms, apart from their obvious appearance in faeces, include anal itching specially at night, a dry cough, constant nose-picking, restlessness at night, dry lips during the day and wet lips at night, and a generally unwell feeling. The child may wake up in the morning with a little pool of saliva on the pillow. Symptoms may even include convulsions or fits. There is absolutely no point in working on the effect without getting right down to the cause, so look first to diet. Cut out all starch including flour, bread and potatoes. Cut out all meat and sugar.

Concentrate on fruit, especially cranberries, papaya and pineapple, seeds, particularly pumpkin, watermelon and cucumber seeds, and vegetables. Include lots of onions and garlic in the diet, which worms hate.

Mix equal quantities of the following herbs together:

>   wormwood (*Artemisia absinthium*)
>   rue (*Ruta graveolens*)
>   peppermint (*Mintha piperita*)
>   male fern powder (*Felis mas*)

Hide this remedy in an electuary as it doesn't taste great, and give an appropriately tailored dose according to the age of the child, night and morning, for three days. On the fourth day give the following tea, having allowed the child only stewed cranberries and pumpkin seeds for breakfast (both of which worms hate):

>   2 parts vervain (*Verbena officinalis*)
>   1 part turkey rhubarb (*Rheum palmatum*)
>   ½ part aloe vera (*Aloe vera*)
>   1 part ginger (*Zingiber officinale*)
>   1 part peppermint (*Mintha piperita*)

Give an appropriate amount of tea according to the age of the child and given the fact that the correct adult dose is one cup three times over the course of the day. Try to discourage the child from scratching the anus by pinning the sleeves of pyjama tops or nightie together with safety pins at the wrist end if the sleeves are long enough. If not, get the child to wear cotton gloves in bed at night until the worms are gone. If the worms are proving particularly stubborn, give a goat's milk enema with a tiny pinch of crushed garlic in it, about ⅛th of a clove to ½ pint milk.

If its tapeworm you're treating, ensure the whole head comes out by sitting the child over a potty of hot milk. I know this sounds silly, and indeed I remember thinking so when I was training as a student and was told this. But tapeworms will only emerge if the atmosphere outside is warm and moist and if there's a prospect of food. I've actually seen a tapeworm detach itself from the body using this method.

First aid measures for accidents and injuries

All these remedies are also suitable for adults.

Bites

Always have a bottle of Dr Bach's Rescue Remedy easily at hand (see page 203). It is an excellent herbal remedy for the treatment of shock (for supplier see page 203). It is particularly effective for children and works very quickly when the child is in shock. Emily, a friend of mine, got bitten by a dog when she was eight while out walking, and we rushed her home and gave her the Rescue Remedy, a few drops in a little water. I thought she would be mortally afraid of dogs after that nasty experience, but by her tenth birthday she was asking for one of her own!

If the skin has been broken by a poisonous snake or an insect, suck out the poison and spread a paste of crushed garlic and vaseline over the wound. After half an hour wash it off with plenty of salt water, then chew more or less any green leaf to a pulp and spread it, spit and all, over the wound, securing it with a cold, wet cotton bandage. Ground ivy, plantain or cabbage are particularly good. Renew the dressing several times a day and wash the wound with an infusion of crushed, strained garlic.

Insects

If it's a bee or wasp sting, don't pick it out, flick it with the thumb nail and the barb will come out cleanly without tearing the skin. If you have it to hand, rub the area with fresh garlic or onions or pulped plantain. Take one teaspoon of echinacea every two hours if you're the sort of person who reacts badly to stings. Adjust a child's dose appropriately.

Apply essential oil of rosemary, lavender and wormwood, two drops of each in a teaspoon of almond oil, once the first fierce pain has subsided a bit. This is a good insect repellant oil and smells much nicer than citronella oil which is commonly used as a substitute. If you don't like the oily feel on the skin, dilute the essential oil in alcohol which will act as a dispersant.

Burns

My American teacher got such a severe burn on his hand that the hospital suggested a skin graft. He healed himself by fasting and drinking copious quantities of carrot juice, and by using comfrey, honey and wheatgerm poultice. The proportions were three parts of powdered comfrey root to half part of runny honey, and half part of wheatgerm oil. The poultice was left on undisturbed and merely added to, so that it not only protected the skin but eventually became part of the new skin. Of course all burns have to be thoroughly washed under cold running water first. It often helps soaking a burn in a bowl of ice cubes initially, until the worst of the pain subsides, for a minimum of ten minutes. This minimises blistering.

The gel from aloe vera (*Aloe vera*) is particularly effective rubbed directly onto a burn and, to a lesser degree, houseleek juice (*Sempervivum tectorum*) also helps. Both are undemanding plants to grow in pots at home, though aloe can grow to quite a size. A mixture of wild lettuce and valerian in equal quantities will help with the pain of the burn if it is prolonged, but cold running water or ice cubes should be your first answer.

Cuts

If the cut is very deep, or blood actually spouts from it, as opposed to leaking or dribbling, get to a doctor as soon as you can. Meanwhile, to stem any bleeding, slap on lots of cayenne pepper externally over the wound and drink half a level teaspoon of cayenne pepper stirred into half a cup of hot water. If necessary, apply a tourniquet.

Once the bleeding has stopped, disinfect the wound with freshly pounded rosemary, yarrow or plantain. Apply as a poultice and keep in place with a cotton bandage. Refresh the dressing several times daily. Once there's a scab over the cut, prevent scarring by applying vitamin E oil directly to the skin.

Nosebleeds

Apply ice cubes over the back of the neck. Pound up some yarrow leaves. Roll them into a ball and gently put into the bottom of the nose. Don't put it so high up into the nose that the child may inhale it into the lungs. Gently extract once the bleeding has stopped. If the bleeding is copious, give half a teaspoon of cayenne in a cup of warm water to drink.

Poisons: from food

First administer an enema if the child doesn't already have

copious diarrhoea and if the food was ingested more than four hours previously. Almost certainly food will be the last thing on her mind, but do ensure only purified water is drunk with a squeeze of fresh lemon juice added. The more the better. Try to get her to control the pain of stomach cramps by deep breathing, using the diaphragm in such a way that the stomach lifts. Give equal parts of tincture of echinacea and liquorice in a little water every half hour – dosage to be tailored to the age of the child. Syrup of ipecacuanha can be given to induce vomiting and clear the stomach, but give sips of peppermint tea afterwards to soothe the stomach. In all instances, assist the body to unburden itself of the poison, don't work against it by trying to stop the diarrhoea, for example, with kaolin and morphine. Once the worst is over, give the following formula every four hours and introduce pure fruit juices:

1 part gipsy weed (*Lycopus europaeus*)
1 part yellow dock (*Rumex crispus*)
1 part burdock (*Arctium lappa*)
1 part elecampagne (*Inula helenium*)
1 part dandelion (*Taraxacum officinale*)
1 part oregon grape root (*Berberis aquifolium*)
2 parts catnip (*Nepeta cataria*)

Administer according to age of child in capsule form, or pour the measured powdered herbs into an electuary of honey or tahini.

Poisons: from household substances

If you don't know what the child has swallowed, ring the hospital on the emergency number, describe the container and give all the information you can. They will advise you what can be done immediately while an ambulance arrives. If the substance is caustic, such as ammonia-based cleaning products, **do not** induce vomiting as it will burn the oesophagus further. Plenty of milk will slow its absorption. If the substance is not caustic, induce vomiting by giving syrup of ipecacuanha. Do not use lobelia tincture as is sometimes advised, as this will only speed up the digestion of any of the substance left internally.

Remember to take along the container from which the poison came to the hospital, or if the child won't or can't tell you the source of the poison, take any vomit in a sealed container. Keep the child warm. If she is getting drowsy, give peppermint tea in a double-strength decoction. If she is unconscious, do not give anything at all. Aspirin and paracetamol do not initially induce coma, but in large quantities they do damage the liver, so act quickly and get the child to hospital.

Shock

Dr Edward Bach's Rescue Remedy

This is a combination of the natural essences of five flowers: cherry plum, clematis, impatiens, rock rose, and star of Bethlehem. It is a useful ready-made medicine to have on hand for all emergencies which include shock. If the patient is unconscious, moisten the lips with a few drops or rub some into the pulse points at the wrist. If the patient can drink, give four drops in a little water and repeat very fifteen minutes until the worst is over, at which point reduce to four drops in a teaspoon of water to be held on the tongue for thirty seconds before swallowing, four to six times daily. Rescue Remedy is also prepared as an ointment and can be applied to bruised, damaged or inflamed skin. Both are available by mail order from: The Dr Edward Bach Centre, Mount Vernon, Sotwell, Nr Wallingford, Oxfordshire OX10 0PZ.

Shock can be one of the main products of sudden and sometimes permanent cell changes in the body, and it is one of the major contributors in all disease, which is why I find the Rescue Remedy so invaluable. Have some on hand at all times. It comes in a tiny bottle with its own dropper and is easily slipped into a purse, pocket or the glove box of your car.

CHAPTER 8

Adult Health: Minor Ailments

Some of the ailments I list in this chapter you may consider major problems because you've had to suffer with them personally for so long. Others that I list in Chapter 9 under major ailments you may think of as ongoing nuisances but nothing particular to worry about. Just because it's mentioned in Chapter 9, don't panic and think you're on your last legs. The division between minor and major ailments is fairly arbitrary because so much depends on how you cope with a specific illness. Some minor ailments you'll find in Chapter 7 on children. If you can't find what you're looking for, use the index at the back. Some serious conditions like cancer, multiple sclerosis, and severe mental illness I haven't discussed at all, because they are beyond the province of a book intended for self-help and home use.

For your guidance illnesses are listed collectively under the parts of the body they affect, as in legs, eyes, heart etc, and in each section they are placed in alphabetical order.

Eye problems

Blocked tear duct
Take the calcium formula (see page 258) with horsetail tea. Make a poultice of Fuller's earth and horsetail tea and apply it over the closed eyelid on a thin piece of gauze, leaving it on for twenty minutes once daily. Bathe the eyes with a weak infusion of St John's wort. Ensure that the liver and bowel are working well and get plenty of rest.

Conjunctivitis
The vernal form of this, meaning the type that frequently occurs in the spring, is often due to calcium deficiency, so take the

calcium formula on page 258. Fast for three to four days using carrot juice and assist the kidneys during the fast with goldenrod tea. Bathe the eyes often with freshly made, strained, tepid teas of any of the following herbs – cornflower, mullein, plantain, marigold or eyebright. Take two level tablespoons of rue tea before each meal as long as the condition lasts.

Nose problems

Mucus congestion

Michael Tierra offers the following Ayurvedic formula which acts as a natural antihistamine:

> 2 parts anise seed (*Pimpinella anisum*)
> 1 part black pepper (*Piper nigrum*)
> 1 part ginger (*Zingiber officinale*)

Stir the finely powdered herbs into a little honey and take a half teaspoon three times daily before meals. It tastes very powerful and makes you so hot you sweat profusely. Don't worry, that's what it's supposed to do. Follow a mucusless diet of fruits, vegetables, nuts, grains and seeds only.

Nasal polyps

Follow the advice for sinusitis and, in addition, if the polyps are bleeding, use a tiny pinch of tormentilla as a snuff, remembering to sniff it up both nostrils. Otherwise, paint the polyps with a half and half mixture of tincture of goldenseal and black walnut. You'll need a very fine, thin, camel-hair brush with a slender handle to do this, and it's quite likely you'll sneeze a lot after this delicate operation. Don't worry and do persist. I've treated patients with this, together with good bowel and blood cleanses, and helped them get rid of polyps altogether.

Nose ointment

For sores inside the nose or a chapped nose as the result of too much blowing with a cold, apply the following ointment:

> 1 tbsp petroleum jelly

1 tsp powdered comfrey
2 drops each of spearmint, wintergreen and wormwood oil.

Thick, somewhat messy, but very effective.

Sinusitis

Check that your teeth and gums are in good order. Breathe in vaporised oil from sage and hot water twice daily, keeping the eyes closed so the steam doesn't sting. Rub fresh lemon juice externally over the sinuses. Take the following formulation made as a tincture, one teaspoon three times daily. Equal parts of:

plantain (*Plantago spp*)
sage (*Salvia officinalis*)
garlic (*Allium sativum*)
hyssop (*Hyssopus officinalis*)
burdock (*Arctium lappa*)
lobelia (*Lobelia inflata*)

Chew a teaspoon of grated horseradish macerated in cider vinegar and repeat this process three times daily, just before meals.

Personally I find breathing the fumes while grating it almost as effective. Go to bed with a grated onion poultice on the back of the neck. Ensure you have plenty of the vitamin A and zinc-rich foods in your diet. Really stubborn cases of sinusitis will respond well to a month's course of vitamin A (200,000 IUs) and vitamin D (6,000 IUs), vitamin C (6 g) and zinc (300 mg) daily. This vitamin therapy must be professionally supervised.

Mouth problems

Cold sores

If you're constantly prone to these, look to cleaning up the bowels, the blood and lymph systems. Also ensure you have all the following vitamins daily: vitamin A – 25,000 IUs (for a month only); plenty of B complex; 200 mg B_2 and six grams of Vitamin C. If necessary juice-fast for three consecutive days – if you're strong enough to do so. Dab marshmallow powder on the sore externally if it is weeping or bleeding. If it is dry and cracked, apply goldenseal ointment.

Halitosis

To most people halitosis is a fate worse than leprosy. It is partly an indication of the blocked-up sewage pipe inside you and partly of oral bacteria. So tackle the problem from two angles. Firstly, ensure your bowel is clean (see page 141) and that your diet includes lots of natural chlorophyll (the green tips of freshly sprouted seeds, the juice from wheatgrass, dark green vegetables, etc) and be meticulous about oral hygiene – flossing as well as brushing. Mouth washes with lavender, violet or lemon verbena infusions, or chewing a clove, will sweeten the breath, but only temporarily.

Of those people over thirty who still have their own teeth (and one-third do not), three out of four have periodontal disease, that is, diseased gums round the teeth. It is the most widespread disease in the world and is often relatively painless and therefore symptomless until it is well advanced. The first sign is bleeding gums, which most people tend to ignore, imagining it to be the result of overzealous toothbrushing. Don't be deceived. Get to your dentist immediately, and ask to be shown how to both brush and floss your teeth correctly. If left unchecked you'll inevitably lose your teeth.

Mouth ulcers

Rub the sore with the following lotion:

> 6 drops essential oil of coltsfoot (*Tussilago farfara*)
> 3 drops tincture of myrrh (*Commiphora myrrha*)
> ½ tsp runny honey

Rinse with 1 tsp tincture of white oak bark and 1 tsp cider vinegar diluted in some water. Take a month's megadose each of vitamin A, D and C under the supervision of a medical herbalist. Gargle nightly with warm sage tea, swishing it well round the mouth before spitting it out.

Chest and throat problems

Bronchitis

> 2 parts horehound (*Marrubium vulgare*)
> 1 part mullein (*Verbascum thapsus*)
> 1 part nettles (*Urtica urens*)
> 1 part elecampagne (*Inula helenium*)
> ½ part goldenseal (*Hydrastis canadensis*)

Take two size '0' capsules every four hours until the worst of the condition has passed. Then two capsules three times daily. Massage the chest externally, front and back, with ten drops of angelica oil in two teaspoons of olive oil. Do this daily using firm, upward, sweeping strokes.

Also check that all five eliminative channels are open and are working properly, paying special attention to the bowel (see page 141). And ensure that the circulation and the thyroid are in peak condition.

Colds

Take a hot bath before bed with a teaspoon of ginger and a teaspoon of mustard in it. Hop out and scrub dry vigorously. Get into bed and drink one pint of equal parts of elderflower, yarrow and peppermint, sweetened with honey and spiced with one teaspoon of ginger. Go to sleep while you sweat it out. If the cold hasn't entirely disappeared the next day, fast and take one gram of vitamin C hourly. Drink plenty of honey, lemon and ginger and with each cup take one capsule of garlic oil.

Hoarseness

Equal parts of liquorice, aniseed and sage. Take half a level teaspoon three times daily stirred into honey. Gargle with sage tea mixed with a dash of cider vinegar. Add plenty of spices and garlic to the diet. Drink an infusion of equal parts of sage, anise, agrimony and ginger, well-laced with honey, as often as desired till the problem clears up.

Head problems

Dandruff
Wash with a mild shampoo diluting 1 tsp in ¼ cup water. Steer clear of alcohol, spicy foods, anything refined, hairsprays, hot dryers and spiky rollers. Make equal parts of the following macerated in enough cider vinegar to cover:

> scabious (*Knautia arvensis*)
> freshly-grated ginger root (*Zingiber officinale*)
> sage (*Salvia officinalis*)
> rosemary (*Rosmarinus officinalis*)
> nettles (*Urtica urens*)
> birch (*Betula alba*)

Strain off and squeeze out thoroughly after two weeks. Section the hair and rub the herbal vinegar into each parting with a pad of gauze. Do this after every shampoo. Massage the scalp with dry fingertips and do your slant board exercises daily (see page 288).

Migraine
Equal parts of the following finely powdered herbs:

> Jamaica dogwood (*Piscidia erythrina*)
> lemon balm (*Melissa officinalis*)
> feverfew (*Chrysanthemum parthenium*)
> rosemary (*Rosmarinus officinalis*)

In the event of an attack, take ¼ level teaspoon stirred into a little plain yoghurt, or if that tastes too revolting, try one of the natural sugarless jams like 'Whole Earth', *not* the standard jams made for diabetics. If the migraine is soothed by applying a cold pack to the forehead, omit the feverfew in the formulation.

Follow a hypoglycaemic diet, that is, eating little and often, ensuring you take some protein every 2 to 2½ hours. Avoid coffee, alcohol and all refined and processed foods. Get a good osteopath to check you have no spinal lesions. Check that the bowel is working properly (see page 141).

Neuralgia

Apply a poultice of comfrey leaves with a pinch of lobelia leaves over the affected area as hot as can be comfortably borne. Keep renewing it until the pain dissipates. If the area is awkward for poultice application (the side of a nose, for example), massage in warmed St John's wort oil, shield the area with a cotton cloth, and then cover with the corner of a heating pad.

Also take the following formula:

> 3 parts hops (*Humulus lupulus*)
> 2 parts camomile (*Matricaria chamomilla*)
> 2 parts lemon balm (*Melissa officinalis*)
> 1 part scullcap (*Scutellaria spp*)
> 1 part Jamaica dogwood (*Piscidia erythrina*)

Take one size '0' capsule hourly until the pain subsides and then two capsules three times daily for three months. Check that your diet is superb.

Persistent neuralgia is the result of nutritional deficiencies and metabolic upsets.

Heart maintenance

Measures to ensure a healthy heart

The following herbal tea tastes delicious and was concocted by Patricia Eltinge specifically to encourage healthy heart maintenance. It supports the kidneys, facilitates digestion, strengthens the heart and, best of all, tastes great!

Make tea with equal parts of:

> roasted chicory (*Cichorium endiva*)
> roasted dandelion root (*Taraxacum officinalis*)
> liquorice root (*Glycyrrhiza glabra*)
> ginger (*Zingiber officinale*)
> coriander (*Coriandrum sativum*)
> orange peel (*Citrus aurantium*)
> whole hawthorn berries (*Crataegus oxycantha*)
> and a dash of cinnamon and cayenne to give it some zip.
> Drink it hot and unadulterated.

.Also take the following precautions:

1. Eat at least one serving daily of the cholesterol-reducing foods: porridge, sweet corn, kidney beans or broccoli.
2. Include plenty of pectin in your diet. The best sources are cooked apples, an ounce of lecithin granules, or a cupful of alfalfa sprouts – these all reduce cholesterol.
3. A serving of one of the oily fish – mackerel, herring or salmon – will decrease platelet aggregation.
4. Put lots of garlic and onion in the diet, preferably raw to reduce thrombus and plaque formation. If this is too anti-social, eat these two foods any way you like except fried.
5. Reduce your alcohol intake to no more than three glasses of wine a day, preferably with meals, or a couple of tots of whisky. No other spirits are permissible.
6. Stop smoking.
7. Cut out salt, hidden as well as obvious.
8. Get down to your normal weight.
9. A diet high in fat and sugar greatly accelerates the risk of heart problems. ***Don't*** go onto polyunsaturated margarine. It is hydrogenated and contains as much as forty per cent trans-fatty acids which raise cholesterol and inhibit the production of prostaglandins, which help lower blood pressure and reduce platelet dumping. Refined cooking oils (that is, those which are not virgin and cold-pressed) are unprotected from oxidation and from forming free radicals which tend to damage artery walls encouraging arteriosclerosis. You're better on a *little* unsalted butter if you must. When using virgin cold-pressed oils, add the contents of a capsule of vitamin E (d-alpha-tocopherol acetate) to the bottle and keep it in the fridge when not in use.

Dairy products are out, except for the odd bit of yoghurt. Include lots of sauerkraut in the diet for its valuable lactic ferment. Important vitamins include A, C, and E; important minerals are selenium, calcium, magnesium, and potassium.

Gastrointestinal problems

Diarrhoea

Remember this is the other side of constipation and means the bowel is heavily encrusted with mucus and needs to be cleared (see page 141). Adults should fast on bananas and slippery elm gruel, and children on strained carrot. Take one teaspoon of tormentilla tincture every two hours until the diarrhoea is under control. Adjust the child's dose according to age. Then follow with a thorough bowel cleanse coupled with rejuvelac (see page 17).

Gastroenteritis

4 parts arrowroot (*Maranta arundinaceae*)
4 parts slippery elm (*Ulmus fulva*)
2 parts cayenne (*Capsicum annum*)
1 part cinnamon (*Cinnamomum zeylanicum*)

Mix the finely powdered herbs and take half a teaspoon hourly in a little plain yoghurt for as long as necessary. If the abdomen is specially sore and tender, apply a warm camomile poultice over the area. Don't eat until the infection has cleared up completely, not even the popular remedy of boiled rice.

Indigestion

Any form of acid indigestion needs to be treated by learning not to swallow air while eating. So food should be well chewed in silence. Forget the witty dinner conversation – if you simply must talk put down your knife and fork and stop eating or drinking while you do so. Learn to food-stack (see page 34). Ensure you're not cooking with aluminium utensils and eliminate aluminium from your life. Hidden in food it reacts badly with alkaline saliva and wreaks havoc in the duodenum, causing all sorts of digestive upsets. It's final accumulation in the body's tissues as you grow older is much denser than calcium. Avoid antacids. I know it's the first thing you'd normally reach for, but they're heavy with aluminium hydroxide which has an alarming tendency to lower the level of phosphate in the blood. Prolonged use of antacids may weaken bones and muscles and certainly won't help your indigestion. It coalesces in all the body's tissues but the brain tends to be particularly hard hit, and Dr Pfeiffer of the Brain Bio Research Centre at Princeton believes it may be implicated in cases of memory loss and slow learning.

So examine your pots, pans and kettles, and if in doubt throw them out and replace with stainless steel, enamel or glass. Use clear baking bags, not tin foil. Don't use deodorants. The purer your diet, the less offensive your body odour. Get your skin working properly for you (see page 149). Filter your water. Don't buy cans or cartons with aluminium lining. Check your toothpaste doesn't come from an aluminium tube, or better still, use a natural toothpaste. Don't use baking powder. Let your dough rise naturally or use yeast.

If you get indigestion, chew a piece of calamus root (*Acorus calamus*). If you're eating a protein meal, sip a glass of pure pineapple juice as an aperitif twenty minutes beforehand. The protopeptic enzymes in it will help to break protein down and facilitate its digestion. In an emergency you can always put a teaspoon of cinnamon in a glass of water and sip it, or sip a cup of anise or ginger tea. To facilitate the production of hydrochloric acid in the stomach, take a digestive enzyme tablet with each meal or begin with a slice of papaya.

Don't try the popular remedy of drinking a glass of milk – this only makes matters worse by depressing the production of hydrochloric acid in the stomach, facilitating the absorption of undesirable elements like lead, and blocking the absorption of vital minerals like zinc.

Indigestion remedy

2 parts anise (*Pimpinella anisum*)
1 part fennel (*Foeniculum vulgare*)
1 part camomile (*Matricaria chamomilla*)
1 part vervain (*Verbena officinalis*)
½ part calamus root (*Acorus calamus*)
½ part peppermint (*Mintha piperita*)
½ part goldenseal (*Hydrastis canadensis*)

Mix the finely powdered herbs in a little honey and take half a level teaspoon every hour until the stomach settles down. It doesn't taste great, but try and chew the mixture well before swallowing.

Poor appetite
If you simply can't eat, try:

1 part calamus (*Acorus calamus*)
2 parts dandelion (*Taraxacum officinale*)
1 part gentian (*Gentiana lutea*)
1 part fennel (*Foeniculum vulgare*)
1 part wild yam (*Dioscorea villosa*)
1 part liquorice (*Glycyrrhiza glabra*)

Make as a standard tincture in white wine and take one tablespoon twenty minutes before meals and repeat the dosage after meals. Substitute ginger for liquorice if you have high blood pressure.

Haemorrhoids

2 parts stonewort (*Collinsonia canadensis*)
2 parts pilewort (*Ranunculus ficaria*)
1 part dandelion root (*Taraxacum officinale*)
½ part liquorice (*Glycyrrhiza glabra*)

Take two size '00' capsules three times a day at meals with a cup of chicory coffee. Use pilewort ointment externally and insert a little on the tip of your finger if necessary. Alternatively, apply an external poultice of spurge. Take a daily cold sitz bath and splash the anus afterwards with a cold decoction of half-and-half witch-hazel and goldenseal. Just a cupful while you squat over a basin, so you can catch it and use it again, as goldenseal is very expensive. Avoid constipation at all costs, and ensure the liver is working well.

Stomach ulcers

Everything I've just said about indigestion applies to ulcers, only more so. A common misconception about stomach ulcers is that they somehow burn a hole in the stomach wall because the stomach is producing too much hydrochloric acid. The problem is precisely the opposite. It is producing too little hydrochloric acid. It is excessive alkalinity, the result of protein putrefying in the stomach instead of digesting as it should do, due to lack of hydrochloric acid that irritates the digestive tract. That is why stomach ulcers go together with heartburn and acid indigestion like the proverbial horse and carriage. So I stress again, antacids are absolutely the wrong thing to take, and I'm certain that a hundred years from now our descendants will look back at the use of antacids with the same pitying horror with which we now regard leeches.

Wherever there is an ulcer or a pre-ulcerous state, the need is for more acid, not less. Don't take over-the-counter drugs which provide a mucilagenous coating protecting the ulcerated tissue. The problem with these is they are too effective, because they actually stop nutrients passing through the stomach wall into the bloodstream, and you sorely need all the nutrients you can get. Make up or obtain the following formulation:

2 parts slippery elm (*Ulmus fulva*)
2 parts marshmallow (*Althaea officinalis*)
2 parts comfrey (*Symphytum officinale*)
1 part angelica (*Agnelica archargelica*)
2 parts poke root (*Phytolacca americana*)
2 parts echinacea (*Echinacea angustifolia*)
6 parts goldenseal (*Hydrastis canadensis*)

Take 2-3 size '00' capsules before every meal, or mix with a little water and take it off the spoon. Also drink three glasses of freshly pressed cabbage juice daily and take as much slippery elm gruel during the course of the day as you comfortably can. Switch to a vegetarian diet with absolutely no coffee or alcohol. Learn, and then regularly practise, deep relaxation exercises. Ensure the lower colon is kept clear. If you smoke, try not to, but if giving up sends your stress levels rocketing, don't swallow your saliva while smoking and rinse your mouth out after each cigarette.

Weakness and emaciation

4 parts alfalfa (*Medicago sativa*)
2 parts ginseng (*Panax ginseng*)
2 parts comfrey (*Symphytum officinale*)
1 part gentian (*Gentiana lutea*)
1 part prickly ash (*Zanthoxylum americanum*)

Make a double-strength decoction using 2 oz of the herb mixture to 1 pt of water. Strain and add the equivalent amount of malt and 1 tbsp black strap molasses. Heat and stir until they are dissolved. Take two tablespoons before each meal. If your digestion is poor, take digestive enzymes too. This formulation will stimulate the digestion, encourage blood circulation and is rich in vitamins and minerals. It will also sustain and strengthen the heart, normalise blood pressure and increase resistance to disease.

Kidney and bladder problems

Oedema (water retention)

2 parts clivers (*Galium aparine*)
1 part dandelion (*Taraxacum officinale*)
1 part horsetail (*Equisetum arvense*)
1 part goldenrod (*Solidago virgaurea*)
1 part camomile (*Matricaria chamomilla*)
1 part juniper berries (*Juniperis communis*)
2 parts marshmallow (*Althaea officinalis*)
½ part ginger (*Zingiber officinale*)

Make a decoction and drink half a cup three times daily. Do not drink with meals at all and switch over to the less watery foods, concentrating on those high in potassium. Apply ginger fomentations over the kidneys once daily.

Retention of urine

4 parts dandelion root (*Taraxacum officinale*)
4 parts parsley root (*Petroselinum spp*)
2 parts buchu (*Barosma betulina*)
1 part uva-ursi (*Arctostaphylos uva-ursi*)
1 part ginger (*Zingiber officinale*)
1 part comfrey root (*Symphytum officinale*)

Make a decoction of the three roots. Make an infusion of the remaining ingredients using freshly boiled water which has been allowed to cool for a few minutes. Mix together and sip one cup, when cool, before each meal.

If the retention of urine is serious, that is, the patient is unable to pass urine at all, call the doctor and meanwhile apply a warm compress of parsley leaves and root over the kidneys.

Back problems

Lumbago

Check that your kidneys are working properly and cut out all tea, coffee, cocoa and alcohol. Take the following formulation:

> 4 parts dandelion (*Taraxacum officinale*)
> 2 parts meadow-sweet (*Spiraea ulmaria*)
> 1 part scullcap (*Scutellaria spp*)
> 1 part lobelia (*Lobelia inflata*)
> 1 part marshmallow (*Althaea officinalis*)

Make a decoction and take half a cup every three hours. Make up the following back pack:

> 2 parts marshmallow (*Althaea officinalis*)
> 2 parts comfrey (*Symphytum officinale*)
> 1 part wood betony (*Betonica officinalis*)
> 1 part dandelion (*Taraxacum officinale*)
> 1 part yarrow (*Achillea millefolium*)
> 1 part ginger (*Zingiber officinale*)

Make a decoction and soak a cloth in the strained mixture. Wrap it round the whole trunk extending from under the armpits to the pubic bone. Cover it in plastic to save leakage and retire to bed, protecting the sheet with plastic to prevent the mattress getting wet. The next morning unwrap yourself and sponge down with half-and-half cider vinegar and warm water. Repeat nightly until the attack subsides.

Osteoporosis

Follow the diet for arthritis (page 244). Take the calcium supplement (see page 258) with a cup of nettle and horsetail tea three times daily, the last dose to be taken just before bed. Women should also take the formula to strengthen the reproductive organs, which is rich in natural hormones (see page

275). Exercise is vitally important and skipping is especially recommended for its piezoelectric effect, that is, its effect of generating electricity in the body.

Skin problems

Abscesses

>   3 parts echinacea (*Echinacea angustifolia*)
>   1 part goldenseal (*Hydrastis canadensis*)
>   1 part thyme (*Thymus vulgaris*)
>   1 part liquorice (*Glycyrrhiza glabra*)

Take óne size '00' capsule hourly until the infection subsides then reduce dose to two size '0' capsules with each meal. This will help abscesses anywhere on the body.

Apply a poultice of equal parts of comfrey, slippery elm, and marshmallow, adding a quarter level teaspoon of lobelia. Mix with a little witch-hazel to moisten. Renew twice daily. Ensure the bowel is working properly.

Acne

Avoid all animal proteins, dairy products, refined and processed foods, spices, shellfish and iodised salt. Use toasted and ground sesame seeds which are rich in níacin to replace salt. Also take one B complex and 300 mg of niacin, 100 mg with each meal daily. For one month only, under the supervision of an orthomolecular specialist, take 150,000 IUs of vitamin A. Ensure there is 1 tbsp of cold-pressed oil in your daily diet. Tension plays havoc with the hormonal balance of the body, increasing the two things acne sufferers can do without; oily secretions and perspiration.

Keep your skin sparkling clean and at all costs avoid the temptation of picking at pussy spots. If you have oozing pustular acne, avoid facial steams. Wash with an infusion of soapwort instead of ordinary soap. A little gentle sunbathing helps. Try a charcoal mask too ... Grill a couple of pieces of wholemeal bread until they're burnt to a cinder. Grind to a powder, mix with a teaspoon of Fuller's earth and a teaspoon of clear honey, and spread this thickly on the face. Leave for half an hour, and rinse

off with warm water. Use strained lavender tea to close the pores
and normalise the secretion of sebaceous glands, splashing it on
as a face wash. This mask will cleanse the skin without making it
unbearably itchy or dry, as harsher acne masks tend to do. Do
daily deep-breathing exercises and make sure the colon is open
and working properly. Take the following formula:

> 3 parts echinacea (*Echinacea angustifolia*)
> 2 parts burdock (*Arctium lappa*)
> 2 parts dandelion (*Taraxacum officinale*)
> 1 part elderflower (*Sambucus nigra*)
> 1 part fenugreek (*Trigonella foenumgraecum*)
> 1 part thyme (*Thymus vulgaris*)
> 1 part ginger (*Zingiber officinale*)

Take one size '0' capsule every waking hour till the condition
is noticeably improved, which may take several days, then
reduce to two size '0' capsules with meals till it clears up
altogether.

If the acne is severe you could get your doctor or dermatologist
to treat you with vitamin A topically in its acid form. It's called
Roaccutane and, though very effective, can cause foetal
abnormalities if taken early in pregnancy, so women using it
should be using an efficient contraceptive method, though it
doesn't seem to damage men's sperm. Expect with this wholist
treatment to get worse for 6-8 weeks before you get better.

Bruising easily

A skin that does this needs its venous system strengthening and
high doses of vitamin C with bioflavanoids. Take the following
formulation:

> 2 parts cayenne (*Capsicum annum*)
> 2 parts comfrey (*Symphytum officinale*)
> 2 parts rosehips (*Rosaceae*)
> 1 part chickweed (*Stellaria media*)
> 1 part fenugreek (*Trigonella foenumgraecum*)
> ½ part goldenseal (*Hydrastis canadensis*)

Take two size '00' capsules three times daily with a cup of
rosehip tea between meals.

Excessive perspiration

Attend to the well-being of the kidneys, the colon and the lymphatic system and don't, whatever you do, try to block the skin with talc or creams. Take the following formulation:

2 parts rosemary (*Rosmarinus officinalis*)
2 part lemon or balm (*Melissa officinalis*)
1 part bayberry (*Myrica cerifera*)
1 part ginger (*Zingiber officinale*)
1 part witch-hazel (*Hamamelis virginiana*)

Take one size '0' capsule hourly till the condition improves. Drink three cups of sage tea daily for one week only.

Pruritis

Ensure the liver and the kidneys are working properly. Grated potato poultices applied to the affected area help but, if this is not possible as in *pruritis ani* (itching of the anus), dab the area with an infusion of plantain and goldenseal using a piece of clean lint. Wear white cotton underwear and keep the anus as dry as possible. Avoid sugar and antibiotics like the plague and include plenty of iron, calcium and vitamins A and B in the diet. Don't scratch, however great the temptation, and for a few months, while the condition heals, avoid all strong flavours, even herbal ones like cayenne, mustard or horseradish.

Roseola (Excessive redness)

This condition is caused by congestion of the capillaries and can be soothed by the daily application of a cold poppy flower poultice followed by dabbing the face with lettuce milk. To make lettuce milk take the outer leaves of one wild lettuce (*Lactuca virosa*), purified water, and four drops simple tincture of benzoin. If wild lettuce is unavailable, substitute any other lettuce except iceberg or Chinese lettuce. Wash the individual leaves carefully and put them in an enamel saucepan barely covering with water. Simmer gently for half an hour. Allow to cool, still covered. Strain through coffee filter paper and add the tincture. Store in the fridge. Do not use soap to wash the skin, use a bag of finely ground oatmeal. Don't sunbathe or use facial steam as both will only aggravate the condition. Attend to the circulation with cayenne pepper (see page 201), and include 500 mg of rutin daily in the diet.

Sunburn

A little sun and air bathing is an excellent idea. It gives the skin a real chance to breathe, providing you haven't suffocated it with layers of heavy oil. But prolonged exposure to the sun causes permanent irreversible damage to the skin. Apart from ageing it, drying it up and encouraging thread veins, it heightens one's susceptibility to skin cancer. If you have overdone it, the following remedies will help:

Cucumber juice – chop it up into cubes, skin and all, put it in a liquidiser and add a couple of icecubes, liquidise, strain through coffee filter paper.

Strong cold tea.

Live plain yoghurt. Messy, smelly but effective.

Neat cider vinegar.

The juice of house-leek as for cucumber juice.

Thread veins

Don't continue to do the sort of thing that started them in the first place, that is, exposing the skin to sudden changes in temperature, drinking tea, coffee, alcohol, working in excessively smoky rooms, taking saunas or eating very spicy foods. Wash the face in lukewarm water only and follow the advice for roseola. In addition, use a very good moisturiser over a skin still left slightly damp with lettuce milk. Nelson's and Weleda make a very good marigold (Calendula) cream which actually helps to heal this condition. Poultices of marigold petals will also help.

Glandular problems

Goitre

Equal parts of:

> watercress (*Nasturtium officinale*)
> kelp (*Macrocytis pyrifera*)
> dulse (*Fucus*)
> Irish moss (*Chondrus crispus*)

Icelandic moss (*Cetraria islandica*)
parsley (*Carum petroselinum*)

Take one size '0' capsule three times daily, the first dose on an empty stomach on rising with a cupful of honey, cider vinegar and warm water. Apply mullein and lobelia poultices over the thyroid at least once daily. Dr Vogel recommends a cabbage and clay poultice moistened with oak bark decoction, but warns that it may have a very strong effect. So leave it on for only as long as it is bearable. If it burns or itches, take it off immediately. Provided this treatment is faithfully followed, it will greatly improve a goitre condition.

Sluggish thyroids

Take the above formulation together with the mullein and lobelia formulation on page 195, leaving a five-minute gap between capsules. Apply a warm mullein and lobelia poultice over the thyroid and leave it on all night. Keep this treatment up until the thyroid has improved and for at least three months. An iridology test will determine how healthy the thyroid has become.

Feet

About seventy-five per cent of us suffer from foot disorders, of which we may not be conscious simply because we do not realise that pain in the legs, back, neck, or head may be the result of a foot disorder. The weight of the body should be borne on the outside arch of the foot which is made of bone so it can do just that. The soft, inner arch is made of ligaments and muscles, and when we stand or walk badly the weight is thrown on the arch, eventually resulting in collapse.

We walk about eight miles a day on average just going about our ordinary business, so it's worth protecting the feet at an early age. Children should have well-made lace-up shoes with rounded toes, with at least the width of an adult's thumb to grow into. Everyone's socks should always be roomy and not crush the toes. Shoes and socks should be made of natural materials so that the feet can breathe easily. In the summer, feet should be bare as much as possible, or sandals should be well ventilated, and socks should of course be changed daily and feet washed and thoroughly dried at least once daily.

Jogging on hard surfaces like pavements and roads really jars the feet and ankles, and overzealous joggers may give their feet such a pounding that the tissues in the feet simply collapse, resulting in arthritic pain and damaged Achilles tendons. So try to jog on grass or soil and don't stint when you buy running shoes. Get them professionally fitted.

Tired, aching feet at the end of the day may point to lack of exercise. Barefoot walking on grass or sand will certainly help, followed by a good self-massage of the feet using rosemary or lavender oil diluted with almond oil, followed by a foot soak in lady's mantle, comfrey or geranium with a dash of cider vinegar. Cold feet can be warmed by sprinkling the socks with cayenne.

Athlete's foot

Wash with a decoction of soapwort and rinse with diluted cider vinegar. Keep the feet scrupulously dry and allow them as much air and sun as possible, but be considerate about walking around barefoot in public places – athlete's foot is highly infectious. Soak your feet nightly in a decoction of equal parts of sage, red clover, agrimony and marigolds with a dash of cider vinegar. Having dried the feet thoroughly, powder them liberally with arrowroot.

Brittle nails

Take the calcium formula with a cup of horsetail tea three times daily (see page 258). Drink honey and cider vinegar and paint the nails with fresh lemon juice. Put on a pair of cotton-lined gloves before tackling jobs that involve the use of detergents.

Corns

Macerate 30 g (1 oz) of ivy leaves and the same quantity of celandine leaves in enough cider vinegar barely to cover. Leave to stand for a fortnight and top up with vinegar from time to time if necessary. Fork out some of the leaves and bind them onto the corn with a piece of linament and a bandage. Change the dressing twice daily. The corn will gradually get soft enough to lift out.

Maurice Mességué recommends a clove of crushed garlic

applied to the corn. Protect the surrounding skin with Vaseline or Elastoplast.

Gout

Take a series of short fasts lasting three days, only using cherry juice. Expect to get worse before you get better on this treatment, as fasting will quickly release all the uric acid into the bloodstream, which may be uncomfortable. If it is, take a blood purifying formulation as on page 145. Then follow the diet for arthritis (see page 244) and include plenty of fresh strawberries and cherries in season. Cut out all animal products, dairy products, fish, peas and wheat, except for sprouted wheat, and drink as much potassium-rich broth as you can (see page 102). Also take:

2 parts sarsaparilla (*Smilax officinalis*)
1 part horsetail (*Equisetum arvense*)
1 part fenugreek (*Trigonella foenumgraecum*)
1 part juniper berries (*Juniperus communis*)
1 part parsley (*Petroselinum spp*)
1 part ginger (*Zingiber officinale*)

Make up as a tea and take three cups daily between meals.

Ingrown toenails

Cut the toenails straight across – not rounded at the corners. Mix alum powder with a little witch-hazel to a paste and spread over the ingrown toenail. Cover with lint and a bandage. Renew twice daily until the swelling and pain are gone. As a preventive measure, scratch the top end of the toenail with an emery board so that it is thin. Do this daily and the toenail will grow out flat.

Leg ulcers

Ensure that all eliminative channels are working properly, as open leg ulcers are nature's way of discharging poisons from the body. Check that there's an abundance of calcium in the diet and take 500 mg rutin daily.

2 parts motherwort (*Leonurus cardiaca*)
1 part St John's wort (*Hypericum perforatum*)
1 part witch-hazel (*Hamamelis virginiana*)

1 part horsechestnut (*Aesculus hippocastanum*)
1 part walnut leaves (*Juglans nigra*)
½ part goldenseal (*Hydrastis canadensis*)
1 part cinnamon (*Cinnamomum zeylanicum*)

Take two size '00' capsules, three times daily before meals. Also apply an ointment made up with equal parts of hydrous lanolin and coconut oil, using equal parts of the following herbs:

marshmallow (*Althaea officinalis*)
slippery elm (*Ulmus fulva*)
comfrey (*symphytum officinale*)

If the ulcers are still open and weeping, apply the above mixture as a fomentation at night and leave the legs open and uncovered during the day.

Phlebitis
Apply a cold compress of equal parts of the following herbs:

witch-hazel (*Hamamelis virginiana*)
arnica (*Arnica montana*)
St John's wort (*Hypericum perforatum*)
yarrow (*Achillea millefolium*)

Stick to a fruit and vegetable diet only until the inflammation has subsided. Internally take:

4 parts echinacea (*Echinacea angustifolia*)
2 parts burdock (*Arctium lappa*)
1 part lady's slipper (*Cypripedium pubescens*)

Take one size '00' capsule every two hours. Once the inflammation has gone, continue the course of capsules for six months but reduce to two with every meal.

Weight problems

Underweight
Underweight is not as rare as you might suppose, confronted as

we are with an avalanche of advice about melting the solid flesh. Nearly thirty per cent of women in their twenties are underweight; thirty-five per cent of women in their thirties. Not all of them have diagnosable anorexia nervosa by any means.

A word of caution here: if you're underweight according to the insurance charts but look great, feel terrific and have bags of energy, you've got absolutely nothing to worry about. But if you tire readily, are highly strung and become easily ill, it's time you put on some weight. This means a diet rich in whole grains and pulses with a reasonable amount of cold-pressed oils and natural sweets like halva, and nuts and seed cereal bars. It's quality you want not quantity, so don't get side-tracked by the banana split. Go for lentil soup with wholemeal bread and butter. Refined sweets and carbohydrates rob the appetite and displace the foods that really count. Half a cup of nuts daily will help you put on nearly a pound a week as they're 400 calories. Half a large avocado is 185 calories, and you can bump that up with a delicious vinaigrette dressing.

Finally, if you're hyperactive, learn to calm down. It'll help you digest your food properly. Don't neglect your exercise; it will help put the weight on in the right places. The following formulation will also help with digestion and ensure the proper distribution of nutrients through the bloodstream:

> 3 parts papaya seed (*Carica papaya*)
> 1 part wild yam (*Dioscorea villosa*)
> 1 part fennel (*Foeniculum vulgare*)
> 1 part catnip (*Nepeta cataria*)
> 1 part gentian (*Gentiana spp*)
> 1 part cayenne (*Capsicum annum*)

Take two size '0' capsules at the beginning of each meal with sips of unsweetened pineapple juice. Also ensure your diet is rich in foods containing zinc (see pages 45 and 105).

Overweight

Attributing overweight to overeating is hardly more illuminating than ascribing alcoholism to overdrinking. The main cause of overeating is a disordered appestat mechanism. In the hypothalamus gland there are two food consumption mechanisms – the hunger and the satiety centres. Dr Roger Williams believes it is possible that an impaired appestat mechanism can be induced in the foetus by poor prenatal nutrition. But this doesn't have to be a lifelong handicap.

Meals should be small and often to correct this (gorging on one big meal a day increases the cholesterol and phospholipid levels). Appestat function can be disrupted by negative emotions too – self-loathing, anxiety, fear, jealousy – so it is incredibly important to correct this and to approach the whole problem of weight loss gently on a psychological level. Warning, threatening and shaming overweight people only sends their own sense of self-worth plummeting.

Obesity is indisputably the result of increased food intake and decreased energy expenditure, so the answer is less food and more vigorous regular exercise. Exercise can actually cut down the appetite.

Programme for weight loss

1.   Avoid sugar in *all* its forms, natural or otherwise.
2.   Take 2 tbsp of cider vinegar in water before each meal.
3.   Eat five or six small meals of unrefined foods per day. Their frequency will make hunger less probable and small meals minimise the conversion of food into fat.
4.   Add some natural oil to the diet every day. It improves the combustion of food and gives a satisfied feeling after eating.
5.   No coffee, tea, alcohol or salt.
6.   Get out and do something in the evenings which doesn't involve food. If you're anything like me, I don't have time to be tempted during the day, but once I'm home I find it easy to nibble.
7.   Take 2 tbsp lecithin daily and the formulation to assist the thyroid on p. 223.
8.   Don't skip meals. If you do so, the resultant fat that pours into the bloodstream rises to six times more than normal, which is burdensome for the heart.
9.   Start an exercise programme and stay with it. Skin scrub twice daily.
10.   Learn to love and value yourself and get the support of someone both knowledgeable and sympathetic behind you, who doesn't have tunnel vision about the basic high

protein diet which seems to be the only way Westerners think of losing weight.

Ensure the bowel, kidneys and liver are working properly **before** going on a prolonged diet. Use blood purifiers and kidney cleansers in the last stages of a diet to help you get over the final hump. In the meantime take the following formulation:

2 parts chickweed (*Stellaria media*)
1 part kelp (*Fucus*)
1 part black walnut leaves (*Juglans nigra*)
1 part alfalfa (*Medicago sativa*)
1 part horsetail (*Equisetum arvense*)
1 part plantain (*Plantago spp*)
1 part Irish moss (*Chondrus crispus*)
1 part turkey rhubarb (*Rheum palmatum*)
1 part cinnamon (*Cinnamomum zeylanicum*)

Take two size '0' capsules twenty minutes before each meal with a cup of dandelion tea or coffee. This will support the thyroid, help to cleanse the colon, kidneys and liver, boost the metabolic rate and ensure a correct sodium/potassium ratio.

General spring clean

I feel everyone who is capable of doing so would benefit from a short fast at the turn of each season, but spring is a particularly important time of the year for getting rid of winter stodge and gearing up a sluggish body to full throttle again.

Fast for three or four days on juice of your choice. Then go onto a further three days of fruit and vegetables only, with added plain yoghurt if desired. Take the following formulation for three weeks only. Equal parts of:

angelica (*Angelica archargelica*)
burdock (*Arctium lappa*)
yellow dock (*Rumex crispus*)
echinacea (*Echinacea angustifolia*)
nettles (*Urtica urens*)
chickweed (*Stellaria media*)
senna (*Cassia angustifolia*)
dandelion (*Taraxacum officinale*)

cayenne (*Capsicum annum*)

Take three size '00' capsules in the morning and three at night with a cup of red clover tea. Omit the angelica if you are hypoglycaemic or pregnant.

CHAPTER 9

Adult Health: Serious Ailments

It has been said that allopathic medicine is well equipped to handle the terminal or catastrophic diseases like cancers, sclerotic heart diseases, arthritis – by writing out death certificates. My own view is somewhat less harsh. If we practised true preventive medicine, such diseases would not have swelled to their current epidemic proportions but, given the fact that we don't, the people who suffer from them should at least be allowed an informed choice as to the various ways in which their condition could be treated – chemically, nutritionally, biologically, spiritually.

I am happy to see what has been dubbed the Bristol method becoming at least widely known, if not yet widely accepted. At the centre in Bristol people with so-called terminal cancers are encouraged to take responsibility for their own well-being and use every method available to them to get well. Some may choose to integrate allopathic medicines into a regime which is essentially natural, while others plump for the natural path only. Either way they do so fully informed about the side-effects of both. And that's what I find so heartwarming. Essentially it is an informed approach in which the patient is allowed to make the decisions about their own body. Getting well, whether it be from a minor or major ailment, is a learning process and, unless we are prepared to participate fully and intelligently in that process, we cannot hope to raise our consciousness and so progress.

I am greatly privileged at the moment to be working with a particularly courageous woman who two years ago was told she had two tumours on her liver and was given six months to live. Notice I said 'working with'. I don't dispense cures. I teach people the many ways in which they can help themselves. Once the ball is in their court it's up to them to pick it up and run with it. I'm there on the sidelines shouting encouragement. This woman is still running and it hasn't been smooth going by any means, but she tells me that, given her time again, she'd still choose to tread the same path because she believes her disease has been a terrific learning process, one that has revolutionised her life. Certainly I feel that when her time comes, whatever she dies of, it won't be liver cancer. So you see there are no incurable diseases, there are only people who think they're incurable.

If you have a serious illness, make it your business to find out about all the different ways in which you can help yourself. Question your doctor, your consultant and your alternative practitioner until you feel you've worked out an appropriate path for yourself. Let whoever is helping you know what you have decided to do and why. Hopefully, by marshalling all the informed advice you can muster, by asking for support from those you love, and by equipping yourself with lots of intelligent determination, you'll overcome your problem.

It is not within the province of this book to deal with serious illness by suggesting you'd be wise to treat yourself. The approaches I've used for the major illnesses I mention in the rest of the chapter have worked well for most of my patients, but I wouldn't like to see patients following them without first consulting an alternative practitioner experienced in these matters, because every individual arrives at a disease by a different path. So treatment which works for one person may not be effective for another, simply because it is inappropriate for their particular disease patterns. So use my approaches only for general guidance.

Eye problems

Far too few people visit an optician regularly for a check-up, and yet you should go throughout your life as naturally as you go to the dentist, only not as often: once every two or three years is fine unless you wear glasses or contact lenses, in which case it should be once every eighteen months. After the age of forty you should go every year, regardless of whether or not you wear glasses or contact lenses, because this is the age at which glaucoma is more likely to develop. An optician can spot not just cataracts or glaucoma, but some types of circulatory problems too. Approximately four per cent of the over-forties develop glaucoma, and large numbers suffer severe sight restriction or blindness as a result. Yet glaucoma caught early can be treated very successfully simply by lowering the intra-ocular pressure and keeping it within normal range. Your optician will prescribe drops to do this locally in cases of chronic simple glaucoma, and the following formulation is a gentle systemic way to help back up this treatment.

Formulation to help glaucoma

scullcap (*Scutellaria spp*)
turkey rhubarb (*Rheum palmatum*)
gipsy weed (*Lycopus europaeus*)
gentian (*Gentiana lutea*)
figwort (*Scrophularia nodosa*)
plantain (*Plantago spp*)
angelica (*Angelica archargelica*)
dandelion (*Taraxacum officinale*)
oregon grape wort (*Berberis aquifolium*)

Mix equal parts of the finely powdered herbs and take two size '00' capsules three times daily. In addition to the eyedrops prescribed for you, angelica and eyebright may be used in cooled decoction form as an eye wash. Also take 200 mg of potassium gluconate and 300 mg of nicotinamide (the non-flushing form of B_3) nightly with one B complex – 75 mg. Cut out absolutely all salt.

Avoid eyestrain by taking short rests while reading or writing if you propose to do so for a long time. Improve the muscles and lens of the eye by following the Bates eye exercises daily. Details from: The Secretary, 49 Queen Anne Street, London W1

Meuniere's disease

4 parts of kola nuts (*Cola vera*)
1 part ginseng (*Panax quinquefolium*)
1 part bayberry (*Myrica cerifera*)
1 part white oak bark (*Quercus alba*)
4 parts mistletoe (*Viscum album*)

Make a standard tincture and take fifteen drops three times daily. This formulation should be taken under the supervision of a medical herbalist.

Heart and circulatory problems

Angina

Follow the advice for high blood pressure and supplement the diet with vitamin E, starting with 200 IUs and ascending to 1,600 IUs under the supervision of a medical herbalist, who will check your blood pressure and take close note of your medical history. Couple this with 3 g of vitamin C daily and 2 tbsp of lecithin granules. Avoid emotional stress. In the event of an attack, place warmed poultices of cider vinegar round the top of the arms and keep changing them as necessary, or put the following compress over the heart:

> 1 part hawthorn berries (*Crataegus oxycantha*)
> 1 part celandine (*Cheidonium majus*)
> 1 part sage (*Salvia officinalis*)

Have the mixture ready brewed and closely covered in the fridge and warm it up as necessary. Leave it on for ten minutes until cool and then replace with a warm one. Also take the same formula as for high blood pressure.

Begin creative walking, that is, start with a few minutes and frequent rests on the flat and gently build up till you're walking at a sustained pace for an hour daily. The cumulative effects on the heart's action will soon be noticeable. It was George Macaulay Trevelyan who said, 'I have two doctors, my left leg and my right'. Don't be frightened to use them.

Hardening of the arteries

Detoxify yourself from lead, copper, aluminium, etc (see page 107). Definitely no smoking and follow the advice about diet and exercise for angina (see above). Take plenty of the cholesterol-reducing foods daily: cooked oats and barley, sweetcorn, kidney beans and broccoli. Use daily foot baths of garlic and hawthorn berries equally mixed. Equal parts of:

> angelica (*Angelica archargelica*)
> safflower (*Carthamus tinctorius*)
> sanicle (*Sanicula europaea*)

dandelion (*Taraxacum officinale*)
borage (*Borago officinalis*)
cayenne (*Capsicum annum*)

Take two size '00' capsules three times daily.

Heart attack

Administer 3 tsps of cayenne in warm water initially and then ½ tsp every fifteen minutes until the crisis has passed. If possible, give foot or hand baths of black mustard powder, 2 handfuls to a litre of water while waiting for the doctor or ambulance to arrive.

High blood pressure

A supervised juice fast for three to four weeks is an excellent way of bringing the blood pressure down to normal. Use citrus fruit, blackcurrant, grape, carrot, spinach and comfrey juices, the vegetable ones to be taken with a dash of onion or garlic. A brown rice fast works equally well. However, I must emphasise that such fasts must be done under the close supervision of a medical herbalist or naturopath, as they may not be suitable for everyone and you will need an individual examination to determine this. If you cannot fast, try a watermelon diet for a week, and again please seek the guidance of a professional.

A simple way to regulate either high or low blood pressure is a teaspoon of cayenne in a glass of warm water three times daily. You'll need to build up to this gradually – it tastes pretty fiery. Include lots of garlic, buckwheat (for its rutin content), sprouted alfalfa and raw foods in the diet and avoid absolutely salt, tea, coffee, chocolate, cocoa, alcohol and all strong spices and flavouring except cayenne and garlic. Meals should be small, and weight controlled.

The following formulation will gradually regulate high blood pressure, while strengthening the heart, protecting the arteries and improving the circulation:

6 parts hawthorn berries (*Crataegus oxycantha*)
3 parts motherwort (*Leonurus cardiaca*)
2 parts rosemary (*Rosmarinus officinalis*)
1 part angelica (*Angelica archargelica*)
1 part hyssop (*Hyssopus officinalis*)
1 part nettles (*Urtica urens*)

Mix the powdered herbs and make a tincture using 4 oz to 1 pint of vodka. Take 60 drops three times daily.

Low blood pressure

This is generally the result of nutritional deficiencies and a backlog of poisons in the body. Attend to these and take the following formula:

6 parts alfalfa (*Medicago sativa*)
3 parts hawthorn berries (*Crataegus oxycantha*)
3 parts limetree blossom (*Tilia europoea*)
1 part hyssop (*Hyssopus officinalis*)
1 part cayenne (*Capsicum annum*)
1 part ginseng (*Panax ginseng*)

Take one cup three times daily with meals.

Gastrointestinal problems

Diverticulitis

2 parts slippery elm (*Ulmus fulva*)
2 parts plantain (*Plantago spp*)
1 part fenugreek (*Trigonella foenumgraecum*)
1 part St John's wort (*Hypericum perforatum*)
1 part borage (*Borago officinalis*)
1 part ginger (*Zingiber officinale*)

Take two size '00' capsules with each meal with a cup of chicory coffee. Once there is no more evidence of blood or mucus, or after three months, switch to a thorough cleanse with the lower bowel tonic (see page 143). During the course of this treatment and afterwards eat only fruit, vegetables, nuts, grains and seeds, well chewed.

Ulcerative colitis

1 teaspoon of the outer husks of *Plantago major* in a glass of fruit juice four times a day and blood- and lymph-cleansing formulations (see page 145). Avoid bran, all meat, all spices, salt

and pepper; all dried food, all tea and coffee, all freshly-baked bread, all processed foods and initially all unpeeled fruit or uncooked vegetables. Do not drink with meals.

Once the colon has begun to heal, gradually introduce raw vegetables and unpeeled fruit into the diet. Sprouted alfalfa is particularly recommended because it helps to root out rubbish from diverticular pockets. Finish the treatment by following through with a good bowel cleanse using the lower bowel tonic.

Kidney and bladder problems

Incontinence
Do pelvic exercises faithfully every day (see page 285). Take two hip baths daily of equal parts of vervain, hawthorn and garlic, and while sitting in it, pat the abdomen firmly with the flat of the hand to stimulate the circulation to that area, as incontinence, especially in the elderly, is often due to chronic general debility, that is, being run down all over. (For herbal formulations, see page 216).

Kidney and bladder stones
2 parts corn silk (*Zea mays*)
2 parts parsley (*Petroselinum spp*)
2 parts gravel root (*Eupatorium purpureum*)
2 parts hydrangea (*Hydrangea aborescens*)
1 part borage (*Borago officinalis*)
3 parts slippery elm (*Ulmus fulva*)
½ part ginger (*Zingiber officinale*)

Make a tincture and take 15 drops three times daily. Take also daily 300 mg magnesium, 300 mg B_6 and one B complex 75 mg. Compresses over the kidneys of the above ingredients in proportion also help. If you feel you are about to pass a kidney stone, try if you can to drink several cupfuls of slippery elm gruel and apply poultices of equal parts of slippery elm and freshly minced parsley to the kidneys and over the lower abdomen to ease the pain and ensure the speedy and safe exit of the stone.

Liver and gall-bladder problems

Cirrhosis of the liver

This disease is now one of the ten leading causes of death, so general liver maintenance is a good idea. No refined or processed foods whatsoever, only a touch of unsalted butter – all other fats to be natural vegetable oils – absolutely no dairy products, no spices or pickles. Protein to be from vegetarian sources only and no eggs allowed. Lots of vegetables, especially carrots, cucumber, artichoke, beetroot, radishes and horseradish, lots of grapes, grapefruit and lemons. If you're strong enough to fast, juice fast once weekly and apply castor oil packs to the liver and abdomen. Drink plenty of dandelion coffee. Ensure your intake of the B vitamins, particularly choline, is adequate (see pages 53-65 and 68-70). And, of course, no alcohol at all.

Take the following powdered herbs:

2 parts dandelion (*Taraxacum officinale*)
2 parts oregon grape root (*Berberis aquifolium*)
1 part agrimony (*Agrimonia eupatoria*)
1 part rosemary (*Rosmarinus officinalis*)
1 part wild yam (*Dioscorea villosa*)
1 part gentian (*Gentiana lutea*)
1 part sage (*Salvia officinalis*)
1 part liquorice (*Glycyrrhiza glabra*)
1 part ginger (*Zingiber officinale*)

Take two size '00' capsules daily with a cup of dandelion coffee half an hour before every meal. Externally massage into the liver area five drops of essential oil of rosemary in a teaspoon of almond oil daily.

Gall-stones

For three days eat only fruit and vegetables, especially grapefruit and the bitter wild herbs like chicory, sorrel, and dandelion, dressed with a little lemon juice and olive oil. Also drink at least three cupfuls daily of slippery elm gruel spiced with a pinch of cinnamon or ginger. This is vital as it will line the internal mucous membranes and protect them from any scraping or cutting as the stones pass through later on. On the fourth day squeeze the juice of nine fresh lemons and have ready a pint of cold-pressed olive oil. Fast for the day on carrot juice and at 7 pm take 5 tbsp of olive oil followed by one tablespoon of lemon juice. Repeat every fifteen minutes until all the oil has gone and finish off any residual lemon juice. If you vomit (which is unlikely owing to the cutting down action of the lemon juice) still persist with the treatment. Within twenty-four to forty-eight hours you will pass all your gall-stones. They may emerge whole or dissolve in a particularly messy bowel movement. This passing of stones may be a bit uncomfortable as the intestines may grouch a little, but it is definitely not painful, even if the stones are quite large, because the olive oil lubricates while the slippery elm protects. You may have a bit of griping but it will not hurt as you pass the stones.

Revert back to your fruit and vegetable diet for the fifth, sixth and seventh day, adding plenty of dandelion coffee to it. Then go onto a good wholefood diet for the next three months and take the following formulation to ensure healthy liver and gall-bladder function.

2 parts dandelion (*Taraxacum officinale*)
1 part parsley (*Petroselinum spp*)
1 part artichoke (*Cynara scolymus*)
1 part chicory (*Cichorium endiva*)
4 parts marshmallow (*Althaea officinalis*)
1 part cinnamon (*Cinnamomum zeylanicum*)
1 part lobelia (*Lobelia inflata*)

Take two size '00' capsules with each meal with a cup of chicory coffee or dandelion tea.

Jaundice (Hepatitis)

2 parts agrimony (*Agrimonia eupatoria*)
1 part chicory (*Cichorium endiva*)
1 part celandine (*Cheidonium majus*)
1 part oregon grape root (*Berberis aquifolium*).
1 part horsetail (*Equisetum arvense*)
1 part ginger (*Zingiber officinale*)
½ part goldenseal (*Hyrastis canadensis*)

Take at least three cups of this made as a tea daily while fasting on carrot juice. Ensure the bowels are working properly and if they are not, take a lime flower enema.

Apply cabbage poultices to the liver. Once the skin and eyes are back to a normal colour, continue with the tea and revert to a diet rich in raw salads including dandelion, chicory and artichoke dressed with olive oil, lemon juice, tarragon and garlic. Continue with the tea for at least six weeks after commencement.

Pancreatic problems

Diabetes

I'm appalled by the conventional high protein and fat diet that diabetics are asked to follow and much prefer a macrobiotic approach where food consists of plenty of pulses, grains, sprouted seeds and vegetables with moderate amounts of oil, nuts and fruit, well chewed in a relaxed atmosphere. Meals should be small and often. The problem with diabetics is the quantity they are able to digest rather than the quantity they can eat, so it is best to leave the table with room for a little more so that all food can be properly utilised. Weight must be kept stable. Four out of five diabetics are overweight before the disease is diagnosed and, in that sense, diabetes is a 'prosperity' disease, largely the result of systematic overeating of refined foods. It is unknown in countries where people are too poor to overeat.

Food should be taken raw as far as possible, as this stimulates the pancreas and increases insulin production. Garlic, onions, carrots, parsnip and whey are particularly recommended, as is a tea made from the pods of kidney beans, which is an excellent natural substitute for insulin because it is very rich in silica and various hormones closely related to insulin. A cup of this tea is the equivalent of one unit of insulin, and three cups, spaced throughout the day, should be taken regularly. Please note that the gradual withdrawal of synthetic insulin and other related drugs should always be carried out under the close supervision of a medical herbalist experienced in these matters. It is possible to rectify diabetes using natural means, but it takes time and persistence.

Vitamins which may need to be added to the diet include

vitamin E to prevent the insidious side-effect of gangrene, the B complex and 500 mg of C to stop diabetic retinopathy, to prevent damage to small blood vessels and arteries and to improve glucose tolerance, coupled with lots of kelp and other thyroid-strengthening herbs and vitamin A, because diabetics have problems converting carotene into vitamin A, as diabetes affects the bile which needs to be particularly healthy for its correct assimilation.

The following formulation will help with diabetes and gradually reduce the need for insulin:

3 parts dandelion (*Taraxacum officinale*)
2 parts fenugreek (*Trigonella foenumgraecum*)
1 part mugwort (*Artemisia vulgaris*)
1 part liquorice (*Glycyrrhiza glabra*)
1 part yarrow (*Achillea millefolium*)
1 part lemon balm (*Melissa officinalis*)

Take 2-3 cups of the tea daily. If you have high blood pressure, omit the liquorice and substitute the same amount of lady's mantle (*Alchemilla vulgaris*).

A forceful hot shower held over the abdominal area should be taken three times daily for ten minutes each time to stimulate the secretion of insulin. Adequate exercise is also important.

It seems that diabetes is more prevalent in soft water areas, so diabetics should drink hard, heavily mineralised water and, if it doesn't occur naturally, they should drink bottled spring water. Chromium and manganese are particularly important for effective glucose utilisation.

Please note: under no circumstances should a diabetic fast. Juices, particularly cucumber, onion and garlic, can be included in the daily diet because they contain a hormone needed by the cells of the pancreas in order to produce insulin.

Hypoglycaemia (low blood sugar)

Meals should be little and often. Avoid refined food, tea, coffee, alcohol, salt and tobacco. Only one teaspoon of honey daily is permissible, and if you can manage without this, do so. All other sugars are out. Eat only one piece of fruit at a time and dilute the sweeter tasting fruit juices half and half with purified water. It is especially important to eat a little protein on rising and immediately before retiring, and protein should anyway be eaten every 2-2½ hours in very small quantities, a few spoonfuls of plain yoghurt or 5 or 6 nuts. The diet should be high in vitamin C, E and B complex. Vitamin E helps store glycogen efficiently in the muscles and tissues, C and B help normalise sugar metabolism. Take 3-4 cups daily of the following tea:

> 3 parts dandelion root (*Taraxacum officinale*)
> 1 part liquorice (*Glycyrrhiza glabra*)
> 1 part lady's slipper (*Cypripedium pubescens*)
> 1 part saffron (*Crocus sativus*)

Ensure there is plenty of calcium in the diet (see page 96), and add at least ½ cup of alfalfa sprouts to the midday meal.

Exercise initially should be gentle and sustained until a noticeable improvement is felt, at which time it should become gradually more vigorous. Gentle walking and lots and deep breathing are the best forms of exercise at the beginning of treatment.

Skin problems

Eczema (see page 191)

Psoriasis

Make sure all the channels of elimination are working superbly well (see pages 143-58). Remember your skin is only a reflection of what's happening inside you. Get plenty of vigorous lymph-stirring exercise, air and sun baths, and skin brush the areas which aren't affected. Swimming in salt water helps but, if you can't do this, add a cupful of cider vinegar to your bath water. Don't wash with soap. Use an oatmeal bag with a handful of marshmallow or comfrey added. Pat yourself dry after a bath, don't rub. Use the following salve on the worst affected places:

> 4 ml plantain oil (*Plantago spp*)
> 2 ml comfrey oil (*Symphytum officinale*)
> 2 ml lavender (*Lavandula officinalis*)
> 100 ml olive oil, virgin, cold-pressed

50 ml wheatgerm oil.

Shake well together and rub in gently over affected areas. It will also help a little with the itching.

Fasting helps enormously but, as it is necessary to undertake prolonged fasts to make any improvement, these must be done under qualified supervision. Four weeks of fasting followed by a two-month gap, then repeat if necessary.

The diet must be a mucus-free one with at least 2 tbsps of virgin cold-pressed oil in it daily. Supplements should include kelp, 3 g vitamin C, vitamin E up to 1,200 IUs, and an initial course of a megadose of vitamin A for one month only. Citrus juices should be avoided, at least until there is some radical improvement in the diet.

Jill Davies has had great success with the following tisane:

3 parts agrimony (*Agrimonia eupatoria*)
2 parts chickweed (*Stellaria media*)
2 parts dandelion (*Taraxacum officinale*)
1 part elderflower (*Sambucus nigra*)
1 part scullcap (*Scutellaria spp*)
2 parts burdock (*Arctium lappa*)
1 part yellow dock (*Rumex crispus*)
1 part plantain (*Plantago spp*)

Drink three cups daily between meals.

Shingles

1 part wild lettuce (*Lactuca virosa*)
1 part vervain (*Verbena officinalis*)
1 part scullcap (*Scutellaria spp*)
2 parts Jamaica dogwood (*Piscidia erythrina*)
2 parts nettles (*Urtica urens*)
1 part damiana (*Turnera diffusa*)
2 parts parsley (*Petroselinum spp*)

Take two size '0' capsules hourly every waking hour till the pain and itching subsides, drinking each dose with sips of dandelion coffee. Jill Davies uses the following essential oil mixture externally for shingles:

2 ml wintergreen oil (*Gaultheria procumbens*)

1.5 ml camomile oil (*Matricaria chamomilla*)
1.5 ml rosemary oil (*Rosmarinus officinalis*)
1.5 ml lavender oil (*Lavandula officinalis*)
1.5 ml thyme oil (*Thymus vulgaris*)

Dilute with 250 ml distilled water and apply directly to the shingles as often as necessary.

Arthritic and rheumatic problems

Programme for arthritis and rheumatism

The main thing is not that the path to recovery is long and arduous, for in my experience it undoubtedly is, but that recovery is possible. Arthritis and rheumatism are curable, contrary to what you may have been told. But everything depends on you. The time it takes depends on how long you've had the illness and, if it is chronic, it may take a couple of years of dedicated application.

Diet

Stick rigidly to a diet abundant in vegetables, their freshly pressed juices, fruit, especially fresh pineapple, nuts, grain and seeds, particularly sprouted ones. Use honey, maple syrup, and black strap molasses as sweeteners, and kelp as flavouring. If it isn't part of that list, don't eat it. Begin each morning with a glass of freshly expressed potato juice diluted with a little water. Drink at least one mug of potassium broth daily. This is easily made by boiling unpeeled, scrubbed potatoes, carrot, beetroot, celery, turnips, cabbage and their leafy green tops where appropriate. Half the quantity should consist of potatoes, the remainder of equal parts of the other vegetables. Include plenty of the iron-rich foods in your daily diet (see page 99).

Fasting

Repeated vegetable juice fasts of four to six weeks using carrot, beet, parsley, alfalfa, potato and celery juices are particularly recommended but this must be done under supervision. Initially the condition may worsen as uric acid floods into the bloodstream. Don't panic and keep at it. Leave an eight week break between fasts and go back on the above diet.

Hydrotherapy

Hot/cold showers and skin scrubbing should be carried out once or twice daily. If you're too poorly to do it yourself, get someone to do it for you. Take Epsom salt baths twice weekly. Massaging painful joints underwater using baking powder is also helpful. Movement underwater in a warm swimming pool is useful too.

Barefoot walking

Do this on sand or grass for a minimum of fifteen minutes a day. If you can't walk, get someone to massage your feet daily.

Exercise

Do some yoga daily or, if this is beyond you, do some simple stretching exercises or get a physiotherapist to work out a pattern of individual exercises for you.

Relaxation and visualisation

Work out a routine that works best for you and be consistent with it. Reading Carl Simonton's *Getting Well Again* (published by Bantam) will help you construct a visualisation programme suitable for your own needs. This is a vital part of your programme, because I've observed that an arthritic personality is one that lavishes time and attention on other people but focuses very little on self-care. Arthritis is closely bound up with stress, the type of stress that results from the exhaustion of the adrenal glands, and conscious relaxation will help combat this. Visualisation is simply the conjuring up of graphic mental pictures which gradually work towards correcting the negative mental aspects of any disease.

Massage

A daily massage will soothe and help mobility.

Poultices and compresses

Mustard packs, castor oil compresses, clay poultices, slippery elm poultices with lobelia and cayenne, and pulped cabbage leaf poultices are all helpful.

This formula will stimulate the liver and purify the blood, ensure the correct assimilation of minerals, particularly iron and calcium, and equalise the blood pressure.

Mix together the following powdered herbs and take three size '00' capsules daily with each meal:

4 parts agrimony leaves (*Agrimonia eupatoria*)
4 parts dandelion (*Taraxacum officinale*)
2 parts burdock (*Arctium lappa*)
1 part yellow dock (*Rumex crispus*)
1 part celery seed (*Apium graveolens*)
1 part goldenrod (*Solidago virgaurea*)
1 part cayenne (*Capsicum annum*)
1 part scullcap (*Scutellaria spp*)

If the pain is excessive, also take ten drops hourly of the following tincture:

3 parts echinacea (*Echinacea angustifolia*)
1 part wild lettuce (*Lactuca virosa*)
1 part valerian (*Valeriana officinalis*)
1 part lady's slipper (*Cypripedium pubescens*)

Jill Davies passed on to me the formula for a tisane with which she has had great success. It is a good general remedy for arthritis. Try it as an alternative to the first remedy:

2 parts nettles (*Urtica urens*)
2 parts dandelion (*Taraxacum officinale*)
1 part agrimony leaves (*Agrimonia eupatoria*)
1 part St John's wort leaves (*Hypericum perforatum*)
1 part meadow-sweet leaves (*Spirea ulmaria*)
1 part burdock root (*Arctium lappa*)
1 part comfrey leaves (*Symphytum officinale*)
1 part horsetail leaves (*Equisetum arvense*)
1 part scullcap leaves (*Scutellaria spp*)
1 part sarsaparilla root (*Smilax ornata*)
2 parts devil's claw root (*Harpagophytum procumbens*)

Take three cups daily. The last ingredient makes the tea slightly bitter, so if you can't manage the taste, omit and take devil's claw tablets instead, following the manufacturer's instructions.

Prostate problems

An alarmingly high proportion of men over sixty, some sixty-five per cent, suffer from prostate problems and the sad truth is it is entirely preventable. Impotence has many causes but it is often related to an enlarged prostate, so if this is a problem, see it as a warning of incipient prostate enlargement. A normal-size prostate is about the size of a walnut but, when it becomes inflamed and swells, it puts restrictive pressure on the urethra and you may notice a deep, dull ache in the lower abdomen close to the rectum, get chronic backache, pain during ejaculation, see traces of blood in the urine or semen, or notice that it is taking longer than usual to empty the bladder. Any retained urine will cause cystitis, which in turn affects the kidneys and leads to a backlog of urinary wastes in the bloodstream. A swollen prostate that is neglected can become cancerous.

The prostate also secretes hormones which are fed into the bloodstream and are a contributive factor to general health and well-being. So the herbal approach to this problem must be two-pronged: one to help the hormone balance and the other to cleanse and maintain the bladder and kidneys and reduce the swelling.

Retained enema

You can reduce the swelling by mixing together equal parts of cold-pressed safflower, olive and sesame oil, measuring out two tablespoonfuls, and squeezing 10,000 IUs of oil-based vitamin A and 1,000 IUs of vitamin E into the oils. Put the mixture in a small bulb syringe and squeeze it into the rectum just before bed, retaining it until your next bowel movement. Do this nightly, remembering to rest on the seventh day, until the swelling is alleviated.

Vitamins and foods

Meanwhile eat at least a heaped handful of pumpkin seeds daily. These contain a male androgen hormone and are rich in vitamins A, B, E, F, zinc, iron, phosphorus and calcium. Take 1,000 IUs of vitamin E daily, working up to it gradually, and take a megadose of A and D for one month only, 25,000 IUs of A and 1,000 IUs of D. Take two teaspoonfuls of bee pollen daily, which is rich in natural oestrogens, or the formula on page 275. Continue to take the pumpkin seeds daily as a prophylactic even after the condition has cleared up.

Herbs

Avoid alcohol and sugar like the plague. take the following formula, coupled with the hormone formula above or with bee pollen. Equal parts of:

> goldenrod (*Solidago virgaurea*)
> echinacea (*Echinacea angustifolia*)
> ginseng (*Panax ginseng*)
> juniper berry (*Juniperus communis*)
> marshmallow root (*Althaea officinalis*)
> buchu leaves (*Barosma betulina*)
> ginger (*Zingiber officinale*)

Take two size '00' capsules in the morning with a cup of parsley leaf tea and two at night. This formulation, coupled with the hormonal one above, may safely be used as a prophylactic to keep the prostate healthy.

Self-massage

Lie on your back on the floor, not on the bed. Now draw up your knees until they touch your chest. Don't worry if you can't reach the chest at first. Press the soles of your feet together. Holding them together, push the legs down on the floor as far as you can. Massage the back of the leg behind the ankle using the thumb and index finger on either side in small clockwise circular motions. This area corresponds to the male reproductive organs in reflexology.

Sitz bath

This is especially helpful in acute cases. It relieves congestion in the pelvis and so helps with the pain.

In the evening, run a warm bath keeping the temperature at blood heat and ensuring that the level of water is such that when you get in it doesn't reach above your navel. Add a quart of strained camomile or lemon balm tea. Now sit in the bath for fifteen minutes with your knees bent so only your bottom and feet are in the water. Keep the room warm. When you get out dry briskly with a rough towel and spend a minute or so patting the abdomen vigorously with the flat of the hands.

Impotence

Take careful note of the previous section on prostate problems and follow the advice on diet and vitamins. Your sex drive may also become weakened due to related weakness of the liver, kidneys, heart or brain, so it is always wise to consult a qualified medical herbalist with experience in these matters. Alternatively, you may benefit from counselling, in which case you will be referred appropriately.

Two herbal measures which, besides the ones already mentioned under prostate problems, will help are: one, a nightly garlic friction rub to the base of the spine. Use tincture of garlic and pay special attention to the triangular area round the sacrum. And, two, mix:

> 3 parts damiana (*Turnera diffusa*)
> 1 part kola (*Cola vera*)
> 1 part ginseng (*Panax ginseng*)
> 1 part spearmint (*Mentha viridis*)

Take two size '00' capsules with each meal. Omit the ginseng if there is any suggestion of prostate inflammation.

Herbal help after an operation

Anaesthetics

An anaesthetic tends to leave the bloodstream and the filtering organs like the liver very toxic and saturated with its after-effects. I know how strict hospitals are about allowing you anything other than prescribed medicines after an operation; but if you take the following dried herbs in with you and ask the nurses for hot water you shouldn't have any trouble.

> 2 parts agrimony (*Agrimonia eupatoria*)
> 1 part kelp (*Fucus*)
> ½ part cayenne (*Capsicum annum*)

  1 part red clover blossom (*Trifolium pratense*)
  1 part gipsy weed (*Lycopus europaeus*)
  1 part dandelion (*Taraxacum officinale*)
  1 part burdock (*Arctium lappa*)
  1 part yellow dock (*Rumex crispus*)

Drink at least three cups daily while you are in hospital (more if you have the opportunity) and keep up this treatment for one month to detoxify and cleanse the body.

Surgical wounds

Help the wound by sprinkling a mixture of half-and-half comfrey root and kelp onto your food while in hospital instead of salt. Once the stitches are out and the wound is quite dry, dress it daily with vitamin E oil freshly squeezed from a capsule. Allow the wound to breathe, uncovered, as much as possible. The use of an ioniser will also accelerate the healing of all wounds.

Convalescence

During any period of convalescence drink 2-3 cups of slippery elm daily and take the following formulation. Equal parts of:

  cayenne (*Capsicum annum*)
  dandelion (*Taraxacum officinalis*)
  oregon grape root (*Berberis aquifolium*)
  kelp (*Fucus*)
  nettles (*Urtica urens*)
  alfalfa (*Medicago sativa*)
  St John's wort (*Hypericum perforatum*)

Take two size '00' capsules with each meal. If you don't feel like eating, don't take the capsules, but if you are fasting remember to take plenty of freshly pressed juices. The slippery elm is a superb nutritive tonic and will help to normalise bowel function and soothe any internal inflammation. The powdered herbs will enrich the blood with iron and other minerals, ensuring their proper distribution. It is rich in vitamins too, slightly antiseptic and will stimulate the liver and the kidneys ensuring their proper functioning.

CHAPTER 10

Women

Conception and infertility

We pass on our genetic blueprints to our children and they tend to get scruffier as they go down the line. If you come from a family prone to allergies, asthma or hayfever, it is more than likely that your children will suffer from the same problem. However, it is possible to change this dismally predictable pattern by raising your own standards of health *well before* the baby is conceived. Far better to prepare and prevent than repair and repent!

If you have a particular health problem and you're planning a family some time in the future, pour all your energies *now* into eradicating, or at least greatly alleviating, it. The prospective father's health is just as vital as the mother's. If one or both of you stumbled through your teens on a diet replete with junk foods, or starved yourself to stay thin, or smoked tobacco or took drugs, or drank heavily, or was so glad to escape from blue knees on the hockey field that you gave up exercise altogether, give yourself at least a year to prepare for a healthy conception.

Programme for would-be parents

1. ***Have a full examination***. When I examine potential parents, I ask them to fill out a questionnaire which supplies me with lots of information about lifestyle, diet, exercise patterns, environmental pollution inside and out, and methods of cooking, gynaecological problems, illnesses throughout life and immunity programmes, patterns of family health, digestive, respiratory and nervous disorder, addictions, dental health and a great deal more. This gives me a fair insight into a patient's basic problems which are further expanded by discussion on a

one-to-one basis. I may then deem it necessary to request faeces samples to detect any blood, or a blood sample to check for anaemia, or hair samples to check for aberrant ratios of trace minerals in the body. An iridology test is also necessary to determine constitutional strengths and weaknesses, toxic accumulations and their siting, the levels of acid and catarrh in the body and their whereabouts. A copy of the slides taken of the eyes is kept as a permanent diagnostic reference, or a picture of the eye on video tape is catalogued or stored for future use because, as the body changes, the irises follow suit.

Sometimes in instances of debilitating illnesses, such as alcoholism or coeliac conditions in the case of the potential father, it is necessary to take semen samples and, as this is outside my area, I refer the patients on appropriately. Sometimes I need more complex blood samples to test for blood lead levels or evidence of VD, and again I will refer a patient.

In any case, parents who are keen to produce a really healthy baby are well advised first to have a good check-up by a qualified person with a real interest in and knowledge of preventive medicine. With the supervision of a medical herbalist they could then embark on an appropriate eliminative and corrective programme and make sure the diet is as perfect as possible.

Dr Williams, in his book *Nutrition Against Disease* says, 'if all human mothers could be fed as expertly as prospective animal mothers in the laboratory, spontaneous abortions, still births and premature births would disappear; the birth of deformed and mentally retarded babies would be a thing of the past.'

Allergies are only possible in a weak, run down body, and the potential for allergy in a baby can be greatly reduced by eating a diet which is sixty to eighty per cent raw and so abundantly rich in vitamins and minerals. However, there's no point in wasting such a diet on a chemically and catarrhally blocked digestive track — hence the need for a thorough eliminative programme first before the real work of building the body begins (see pages 143-58). As toxic heavy metal levels like lead, mercury, cadmium and aluminium are now known to jeopardise foetal safety, a detoxification of these is also vital (see page 107).

2. **Smoking** is known to reduce the quality of the sperm and the ova. Don't.

3. **Contraception** If couples are using oral contraception, I generally persuade them to switch to another method for at least six months before a baby is conceived. Among its other drawbacks, it depletes zinc levels in the body. A copper IUD is also undesirable as it leaves too much of this trace mineral in the body.

4. **Alcohol** needs to be cut right down and preferably taken only with meals, because it leaches too many vitamins and minerals from the body. Any long-suffering liver can be disgorged by fasting one day weekly, using a chicory enema and placing a hot water bottle over the liver at midday for an hour while lying down.

5. **Herbs and vitamins** These should be prescribed according to need, but prospective parents would do well to refer back to Chapters 3 and 4. Dr Bayer, a German obstetrician, stated that he'd never known a mentally retarded child to be born provided the father took vitamin E on a regular basis for some months prior to conception. Its level depends on the history of any disease like rheumatic fever and hypertension, and on blood pressure.

Arabs feed their stallions on wild mint to increase their potency, so plenty of peppermint tea might be worth bearing in mind. They also recommend a drink made of powdered roots of the wild orchid (Orchis masculata) sweetened with honey and served well spiced as generally strengthening. This salep was quite popular in this country before the proliferation of coffee houses.

6. **Exercise** Limp, lazy parents tend to produce duplicate children, so build up your stamina and your strength with an exercise programme that has been individually worked out for you, and make sure it is something you enjoy otherwise you won't stick to it. Women should also concentrate on exercise to strengthen the muscles of the pelvic floor (see page 285).

If you thought a programme like that was challenging, once

you receive the happy news that you're pregnant, you'll discover you've only just begun. Nor is the good news an excuse for happy fathers to slope off and stuff themselves with beer and chips. Staying with a healthy diet throughout life makes good sense, but neither parent should allow themselves to become run down between conceptions, particularly if they're close together, otherwise the subsequent babies will suffer.

A Canadian study revealed that nearly six times as many women on an inadequate diet before and during pregnancy had uncomfortable complications including nausea, anaemia, threatened miscarriage, toxaemia or varicosity. The study revealed a particularly striking fact that, although women may *appear* to be healthy in pregnancy on a poor diet, very often the baby is born in extremely poor physical condition.

I would strongly advise all infertile women to have an iridology test to ascertain the cause of their infertility, which will be as variable and as individual as their fingerprints. Too many infertile women are strongly fixated on their reproductive organs when the problem is more likely to be auto-intoxication. The following formula is a good one for cleansing all the organs contained in the pelvic and abdominal area, for purifying the blood, regulating periods, reducing swelling and soothing any vaginal irritation, relaxing the nervous system and killing any parasites, and it is rich in iron, potassium and vitamins B and C. Infertile women should take extra vitamin E, up to 1,200 IUs a day, providing their blood pressure is normal and there is no history of rheumatic fever. Mix equal parts of:

> red clover blossom (*Trifolium pratense*)
> goldenseal (*Hydrastis canadensis*)
> parsley (*Petroselinum spp*)
> dandelion (*Taraxacum officinale*)
> blessed thistle (*Carbenia benedicta*)
> false unicorn (*Chamaelirium luteum*)
> marshmallow (*Althaea officinalis*)
> comfrey (*Symphytum officinale*)
> lobelia (*Lobelia inflata*)
> ginger (*Zingiber officinale*)

Brew as an infusion and drink 3 or 4 cups daily and also go on a good overall body cleanse (see chapter 5).

Pregnancy

Exercise

The best forms of exercise are brisk walking, swimming, hill climbing and horseriding. Yoga is helpful for suppleness. Don't be afraid to really go at it unless there is a history of miscarriage in your family, in which case stick to yoga. One of my patients was a riding instructor and rode right up until the last few weeks of her pregnancy. Her only worry was the possibility of being thrown or falling off, and certainly less experienced exercisers would do well to stick to swimming in the last few months of pregnancy. It was noticed during the Second World War that women railway porters who had to do lots of bending and lifting of quite heavy weights had very easy pregnancies and easier births than their sedentary compatriots. After every exercise session really unwind and relax. This cooling and calming down is just as important as the exercise. Lack of exercise in pregnancy will result in slack muscles, swollen limbs, and encourages varicosity. It will also make it very hard to get back to your original shape after the birth.

Stress

Remember pregnancy itself can be a considerable stress. Emotional crisis, a poor diet, pain, infection, allergies, extreme temperatures, insomnia and drugs all cause stress. Stress also burns up all your nutrition faster than any other factor in pregnancy. So treat yourself to something you really like daily, by which I don't mean a bar of chocolate. Listening to your favourite music, a nice languid bath, a massage, a potter among the hedgerows, a good read, or a quiet daydream. Your happiness is vital for the well-being of your baby. As Juliette de Bairacli-Levy so poetically put it, 'pregnancy should be a daily song of triumph and thanksgiving in a woman's mind and heart'. Prolonged severe stress during pregnancy will mean there is a greater chance of a child who suffers from neurological dysfunctions, behavioural disturbances, developmental lags and generally poor health.

If stress is a problem, eat six small meals daily and, if you simply can't take solid food, take freshly pressed juices frequently, chewing them well before swallowing. Add a piece of ripe fresh fruit to the juice, some wheatgerm, some sunflower, pumpkin and sesame seeds, and granulated lecithin. Put it in the blender and you have a high-powered protein drink. Crunchy and delicious.

Stress supplementations

The more carefully you buy and prepare your food, the fewer supplements you will need, but at times of stress it may not be possible to get all the nutrients you need through diet alone. So add 25,000 IUs of vitamin A and 2,500 IUs of vitamin D, two sustained-release B complex tablets, one after breakfast and one after lunch, 1,000 mg B_5, 6 g vitamin C sustained-release, two with each main meal, and 1,000 IUs vitamin E, provided your blood pressure is fine and there's no history of rheumatic fever.

Support your poor, overworked adrenal glands with the following formulation. Equal parts of finely powdered:

> mullein (*Verbascum thapsus*)
> ginseng (*Panex ginseng*)
> hawthorn (*Crataegus oxycantha*)
> borage (*Borago officinalis*)
> cayenne (*Capsicum annum*)
> ginger (*Zingiber officinale*)
> liquorice (*Glycyrrhiza glabra*)

Take ¼ level teaspoon mixed with a little sugarless jam or juice three times daily. If there are any problems with high blood pressure, omit the liquorice and the ginseng. Take the supplements and this formulation only while under stress and for a few weeks afterwards.

To ground the build-up of static electricity in your body, walk barefoot in the grass for ten minutes daily, preferably in the dewy early morning. Sounds odd but it is very effective, because it calms you down so that literally you feel well-groomed, and once you've come indoors and given your feet a good rub down with a rough towel and put on warm socks, you'll find they'll be as warm as toast in no time.

Diet

I was a bit taken aback to read in a little booklet published by the

BMA that 'nothing very special is required for your diet in pregnancy. It is certainly unnecessary to add much to a diet that is normally well balanced'. The constituents of a well-balanced diet are, as you will have gathered by now, pretty difficult to come by, ungarnished with chemicals or untampered with by the food processors. In addition to which, most people have a very hazy notion of what a well-balanced diet should be.

So begin by referring back to Chapter 1 and then get even more meticulous, because at no time during a woman's life are nutritional requirements so high as when she is pregnant or breastfeeding.

Protein

The entire structure of a baby's body and brain will be largely made from the protein eaten, and of course a pregnant woman has her own protein needs, not least to form new tissue in the uterus and breasts. Protein intake should be at least 75 g daily. Vegan mothers should pay special attention to getting enough combined foods to make a complete protein at any one sitting, pulse and grain, grain and legume, and so on. I tend to find vegetarians and vegans are generally more conscientious and informed about their protein requirements than their carnivorous cousins, so this is usually not a problem. Bear in mind that gelatin (the least complete of all proteins) has excessive glycine which causes a protein imbalance resulting in a slow seepage of essential amino acids in the urine. So avoid it. Also, if you are prone to allergies, it is best to take most of your protein from vegetarian sources (not cheese and eggs) to minimise the risk of passing on your allergy to the baby. High protein foods like meat, fish, eggs and dairy products tend to be more allergenic than combination substitutes.

Oils and fats

Bearing in mind my general advice about fats, you should have one to two tablespoons of mixed vegetable oils daily. A little unsalted butter is also permissible. Use them as part of a salad dressing; don't heat them.

Calcium

The need for calcium rockets in the last three months of pregnancy, and lack of it will cause leg and foot cramps, susceptibility to tooth decay, irritable headaches, and sleeplessness. It may also mean the baby has faulty bone structure and teeth.

It's hard to get ingested calcium to pass into the blood, and doubly so if there's an undersecretion of hydrochloric acid in the stomach (generally the result of years of faulty diet). Lack of fat also encourages calcium to be discarded in the faeces. Dairy products are not the best or even the most effective source of calcium. Plants are by far the best assimilated form of calcium.

> 6 parts horsetail grass (*Equisetum arvense*)
> 4 parts comfrey (*Symphytum officinale*)
> 3 parts nettles (*Urtica urens*)
> 1 part kelp (*Fucus spp*)
> 1 part meadow-sweet (*Spiraea ulmaria*)

All herbs to be finely powdered. Take two size '0' capsules with each meal throughout pregnancy. If you can't get it down because of morning sickness, mix it with honey and take it off the spoon.

Foods rich in calcium include oats, millet, sesame seeds, and most raw vegetables. Pregnant women need 2000 mg daily.

Iron

The baby grabs a very high proportion of the mother's iron in the last two months of pregnancy, so refer back to the section on iron (page 99) and get plenty of it, remembering not to muddle it up with any vitamin E intake. I'd remind you to get it from natural sources, because ferrous sulphate destroys vitamin E at such a rate that it could possibly cause all sorts of unwarranted side-effects. If in doubt about your iron intake from natural sources, use the following formulation during the last three months of pregnancy:

> 3 parts yellow dock (*Rumex crispus*)
> 1 part comfrey (*Symphytum officinale*)
> 1 part burdock (*Arctium lappa*)

All herbs to be finely powdered and mixed. Take two size '00' capsules in the morning and two at night on an empty stomach.

Do not drink tea, coffee, or chocolate at all during the time you're taking this formula.

Iodine
Lack of iodine in pregnancy increases the chance of still births and may lead to other difficulties. Pregnant women can take as much as 3 mg a day and this is best obtained from safe, natural sources by eating Nori seaweed or sprinkling a liberal teaspoon of kelp over every vegetable meal. It tastes terrible over cereal, which is why I'll let you off at breakfast!

Zinc
This is critical to the development of rapidly growing children in order to protect them from malformations and a particularly nasty skin malfunction. Take a supplement of 30 mg daily and use a water filter because copper piping depletes it.

Magnesium and phosphorus
These need to be kept in balance with calcium for reasons already explained on pages 100-1.

   If you're at all worried about your mineral intake, remember you can't go far wrong with a sixty to eighty per cent raw diet rich in fruit and vegetables, particularly sea vegetables such as kelp, laver bread or Nori seaweed, and the additional calcium and iron formulations. Laver bread is popular in parts of South Wales and is readily available there fresh, or kelp may be taken as a supplement (300 mg daily), or a sheet of Nori seaweed (available from health food shops) may be grilled and crumbled over food daily.

Vitamin A
This needs to be taken in temporary high doses if, during your pregnancy, you succumb to an infection or are exposed to a serious illness like German measles. Take 50,000 IUs for eight weeks only, in consultation with your doctor. Fat-soluble vitamins have difficulty passing through the placenta, which means that babies unfortunate enough to be born vitamin A deficient will be particularly prone to infection. So drink plenty of carrot juice during the last month of pregnancy as it is more easily assimilated than fatty sources of vitamin A. And don't

worry. The colostrum you first feed the baby will be particularly abundant in fat-soluble vitamins and will help build up the auto-immune system quickly.

B complex

Many of the illnesses common to pregnancy such as nausea and oedema are often caused by lack of this group, especially B_6, so see page 53 on the B vitamins and get plenty of them.

Vitamin E

A pregnant woman's need for this vastly increases during pregnancy and a supplement will certainly be necessary. Get your doctor or medical herbalist to keep checking your blood pressure on a regular basis while taking this supplement and look again at the section on vitamin E (page 89). Your daily dose should be 800-1,000 IUs but you cannot start with this much if you have blood pressure problems and you must stop if you get toxaemia. Hence the need for constant checks.

Vitamin K

The intestinal bacteria in our bodies generally produces sufficient vitamin K, but because this vitamin dissolves in fat, it cannot easily pass through the placenta into the blood of the foetus. So new-born babies are particularly susceptible to haemorrhage as they enter the first week of life. To protect against this, many obstetricians now inject vitamin K some twenty to twenty-four hours before labour begins. Determine before you go into labour that this will be the case. You won't be in a position to when you are labouring. To ensure your baby gets as much vitamin K as possible in the early days, eats lots of dark green leafy vegetables, especially alfalfa sprouts.

Drugs

The short answer is don't take any, not even an aspirin, if there's an alternative answer. Malformations similar to those caused by thalidomide have been produced experimentally by penicillin, streptomycin, tetracycline and other antibiotics, by many of the drugs used to stop nausea and by viral infections caught early in pregnancy. Antibiotics taken during early pregnancy can also cause miscarriages.

Herbs
Caution: Herbs which should never be taken in pregnancy include nutmeg, rue, angelica, black or blue cohosh, myrrh, mistletoe, juniper berries, pennyroyal, and squaw vine, except under the supervision of a qualified medical herbalist.

Nausea
In my opinion, nausea during pregnancy is the result of a prolonged period of preconceptual inadequate diet, and it is essential to stop it quickly as poor nutrition at the onset may already affect the baby, besides the distress such enforced malnutrition causes the mother. Nausea under these circumstances is nature's way of trying to flush the toxins out of the body so that the baby as it develops within the womb won't be swamped by them.

Nausea and vomiting are worse on rising because it is at this time that blood sugar is unusually low. So a hypoglycaemic diet is advisable, a little protein every 2-2½ hours, and something just before bed. Absolutely no coffee, tea, sweets or sugar in any form, including alcohol, and it goes without saying, I hope, no refined foods whatsoever. Lie in bed and slowly chew a piece of dry wholewheat toast before getting up.

Vitamin B$_6$ sustained-release 500 mg is helpful together with a B complex tablet if you can keep them down. If you can't, you may be able to persuade your doctor to give you injections of 300 mg daily if the vomiting is severe.

Morning sickness formula
To a standard infusion of spearmint tea add half a teaspoon of powdered ginger and a teaspoon of honey. Sip slowly while still lying in bed and if you feel like it eat a dry piece of wholemeal toast. Ginger is wonderful for all sorts of sickness, including travel sickness. If you can't manage the tea, chew a piece of crystallised ginger or suck some cherry stones.

An alternative morning sickness formula consists of equal parts of finely powdered:

  cloves (*Eugenia aromatisa*)
  ginger (*Zingiber officinale*)

goldenseal (*Hydrastis canadensis*)

Take one size '00' capsule on rising with a cup of standard infusion of raspberry tea. Repeat later in the day. Try not to keep this up for too long. If it hasn't helped the sickness significantly within two weeks, revert to the spearmint and ginger formula with a pinch of wild yam added. Prolonged doses of goldenseal may cause the uterus to go into spasm, hence the desirability of small doses only.

Cramps

As these are generally worse at night owing to the slower circulation of nourishing blood to the appropriate tissues, ensure your last meal is abundant in the right ratios of calcium, magnesium, and phosphorus, and when you take your last dose of calcium formula, take 100 mg B_6 with it (see pages 60-2). Try and sleep with your feet slightly elevated. Calcium won't work properly unless it's balanced by vitamin D, and what better way to get it than from a little judicial sunbathing. If the weather is right, expose a well-washed skin which has been lightly oiled with almond oil and a little essential oil of lavender, lady's mantle, or rosemary, for half an hour a day. Pay special attention to the breasts and stomach, and keep your hands and feet covered. Do your deep breathing exercises while relaxing. If there is no sun, take a supplement of cod liver oil, one level teaspoon daily.

Stretch marks

Breast, stomach and thighs tend to be the areas which expand quickly when you put on weight as the result of carrying the baby, and the result can be unsightly stretch marks. Adele Davis in **Let's Get Well** records: 'A friend who developed severe stretch marks during her first pregnancy stayed on an unusually adequate high protein diet supplemented with 600 units of vitamin E oil and 300 ml pantothenic acid daily during a subsequent pregnancy. Although she gave birth to full-term twins, the stretch marks from the first pregnancy completely disappeared, and none formed during the second pregnancy.' So good nutrition pays all sorts of pleasing dividends. A lotion or oil regularly applied will also help. Try the following:

Stretch mark lotion

> 15 gm (½ oz) beeswax
> 15 gm (½ oz) cocoa butter
> 50 ml (1 ⅔ fl oz) coconut oil
> 30 ml (1 fl oz) wheatgerm oil
> 60 ml (2 fl oz) decoction of lady's mantle
> 6 drops essential oil of comfrey

Melt the beeswax in the top of an enamel double boiler. Add the oil in a slow trickle, beating steadily with a wooden spoon. Then add the decoction a few drops at a time. Take the boiler off the heat and continue to stir steadily until the lotion has cooled to blood heat. Add the essential oil, stirring it in well. Decant into a ½ litre (1pt) bottle. Screw on the cap or push in the cork and shake desultorily until the lotion has cooled thoroughly. You have to do this to stop the oil and water phases separating out while the lotion is warm. Label and keep in fridge. Massage into the necessary areas often.

Constipation and diarrhoea

These are best treated by a short juice fast, and if constipation continues to be a problem, use the bowel tonic (see page 143).

Flatulence

Apart from ensuring you're producing sufficient digestive juices by chewing really well and eating lots of vitamin B complex-rich foods, take wild yam (*Dioscorea villosa*) and fennel (*Foeniculum vulgare*) finely powdered in equal quantities. Two size '0' capsules three times daily with each meal. Drink only peppermint, dill or fennel teas with your meals, if you must drink at all while eating (see page 34).

Varicosity

Nearly a tenth of all women get phlebitis or varicose veins either during pregnancy or afterwards. A simple remedy to help avoid this is equal parts of finely powdered:

> yarrow (*Achillea millefolium*)

St John's wort (*Hypericum perforatum*)
Stoneroot (*Collinsonia canadensis*)

Take two size '0' capsules with each meal. Adequate vitamin C and E is also vital.

Miscarriage

If you show any spotting or think you're evidencing any signs of a potential miscarriage, phone your doctor immediately. High doses of vitamins C and E before and during pregnancy help, as of course does ensuring that the reproductive organs are strong and non-toxic. If you have any worries about miscarrying, have the following formulation dose at hand

2 parts false unicorn (*Chamaelirium luteum*)
1 part squaw vine (*Mitchella repens*)
½ part cramp bark (*Viburnum opulus*)
½ part lobelia (*Lobelia inflata*)

Take one size '00' capsule with half a cup of home-made blackcurrant juice with a pinch of cayenne in it every half hour while lying in bed until the bleeding stops. Then hourly while awake for three days. Then two size '00' capsules three times daily with meals for three weeks. The juice can be made by simmering blackcurrants fresh or frozen, it doesn't matter, with filtered water until pulpy, and then sieving. Add honey if desired and freeze in a cube-tray. Decant the cubes into a plastic bag and seal. The frozen blackcurrants can then quickly be unthawed by heating gently.

The beauty of these herbs is that they will not interfere with the natural process of miscarriage if the foetus is damaged in any way, and if the foetus is dead, they should make its expulsion easier.

For easier delivery

Drink raspberry leaf tea daily, and if in season eat plenty of raspberries. Both are rich in citrate of iron which helps to make excellent blood and tones up the reproductive area. If you continue to drink it together with St John's wort in equal parts after the baby is born, it will help relieve the after-pains. If the pain is in the coccyx (the vertebra right at the bottom of the spine), apply a warm poultice of St John's wort to the area, or, second best if it's out of season, get someone to massage the whole spine with essential oil of St John's wort.

Prenatal formula

Equal parts of finely powdered:

  squaw vine (*Mitchella repens*)
  meadow-sweet (*Spiraea ulmaria*)
  black cohosh (*Cimicifuga racemosa*)
  pennyroyal (*Mentha pulegium*)
  false unicorn (*Chamaelirium luteum*)
  raspberry leaves (*Rubus idaeus*)
  motherwort (*Leonurus cardiaca*)
  lobelia (*Lobelia inflata*)

Take two or three size '00' capsules in the morning and the same number at night, beginning six weeks before the birth, not sooner. The formula helps elasticise the pelvic and vaginal areas, strengthens the reproductive organs, and prevents oedema and heart strain so that delivery is easier.

Labour

Don't overload your stomach with food. Juliette de Bairacli-Levy, a well-known and extremely experienced herbalist, suggests fasting just before the labour so that the energy used for digestion can be diverted into labour. She did this herself before the births of both of her children. She also used the fragrance of crushed coriander and the verbena-scented geranium to soothe her. In Malaya cinnamon sticks are burned and the fragrance breathed in by the labouring mother. Soothing herbal teas can be sipped, and massage of the spine with a poppy decoction is said to help, as is a tincture made from the inside of the seed vessel which protects the horse chestnut (Aesulus hippocastanum). As this is narcotic, it must be taken carefully; no more than five drops hourly. Try and have one or the other. Poppy petals are easily dried and horse chestnut can be bought and made up in advance.

Breastfeeding

To enrich breast milk

As soon as the baby is born, reward yourself with a drink of raspberry tea with honey and half a teaspoon of equally mixed clover, cinnamon, and ginger. Spicy and reviving. Then start drinking marshmallow leaf tea which is rich in easily assimilable calcium and so will improve the quality of your milk. Herbs which help increase milk flow are fennel, cinnamon, anise, blessed thistle and vervain. Remember that whatever you eat the baby will ingest through your milk, so don't neglect your own iron and calcium intake. Keep to a superlative diet. Boost the baby's auto-immune system by including plenty of the bacteriocidal herbs in your diet – thyme, sage, garlic, rosemary, juniper berries amd marigolds. Good milk should be thin and should flow easily. Put a little on your fingernail and tilt it upwards. If it doesn't trickle down easily, it is thick. It should smell good, be pure white, almost blue-white in colour, not yellowish or grey, and taste sweet, not salty or bitter.

To thin breast milk

Drink 60 g (2 fl oz) cider vinegar and a tablespoon of honey twice daily and eat lots of summer savoury, hyssop, thyme, and borage. If you can get them fresh, sprinkle them in food and cook with them, but dried is also acceptable in which case make teas of them too.

To thicken breast milk

Eat lots of soupy grains, onions and garlic, and add plenty of sage, blessed thistle, comfrey and clover to the diet.

Sore nipples

Pound up a handful of lady's mantle leaves or violet leaves to a fine mulch or hydrate a tablespoon of the dried herbs by soaking for twenty minutes in just enough hot water to cover. Add enough runny honey to form a poultice. Spread over the nipple and cover with gauze, a square of plastic and a soft nursing bra. Keep nipples supple by oiling them or applying a little buttermilk or honey.

Inability to produce milk

False unicorn mixed with other glactogogues is believed to encourage the flow of breast milk and a baby's frequent sucking action certainly helps. I've read that some Sicilian women who have never had babies can induce the flow of milk by putting drops of goat's milk onto the nipple whenever the baby is about to give up sucking at what initially is a breast that cannot produce milk. After patiently persisting with this for two weeks, their own milk begins to flow. I certainly think it's worth a try if you do have a baby and can't breastfeed but desperately want to.

Weaning

If you can, nurse for eighteen months until the baby has cut eye teeth, which is a signal that the gastric juices have begun to flow. Babies breastfed for at least six months are known to have far fewer allergies than those bottle fed. Wean the baby gradually, as the comfort of breastfeeding is not easily forgone. Drink copious amounts of cold sage tea to dry up your own milk, and if the baby is fretful and keeps demanding the breast, make a poultice of an ounce of freshly ground, finely milled pennyroyal mixed with an equal quantity of myrrh. Mix with a little purified water, and spread over the nipples. Let the baby suck on that. It will rapidly reduce her desire to suckle, but in this way coming off the breast won't be so traumatic for her.

Alternatives to breast milk

Breast milk is obviously best, particularly if you've made the right food choices before and during pregnancy. It is easily digested, contains antibodies and white blood cells, enabling the baby to fend off disease, contains adequate amounts of iron and zinc (once thought to be deficient in breast milk), and a thyroid hormone which the baby is unable to produce for herself.

However, if you can't feed your baby yourself, steer clear of cow's milk, dried in a formula or fresh. It is one of the most common allergy foods, and was, after all, designed for a calf weighing 80 lbs and mushrooming to 1,000 lbs very quickly, which eats grass all day and digests it in five stomachs. A far cry from your own baby's anticipated development. Try goat's milk instead which is now available frozen in some supermarkets and health food shops. The fat content and the size of the fat globule itself is similar to breast milk. (The fat globule in cow's milk is enormous by comparison, and its fat content four to five times higher.) Besides which, goat's milk is digested in the stomach for only twenty minutes, whereas cow's milk lingers for two hours. Common allergic reactions of babies to cow's milk include excess mucus, skin rashes, frequent colds, diarrhoea, colic or constipation.

Do not feed your baby soya milk alone as it is deficient in iron and calcium and therefore not balanced enough for your baby's needs. By all means mix it with breast milk or goat's milk which will help you achieve a healthier balance. The processed variety of soya milk is even more suspect as it is usually laced with sugar, corn syrup and salt, so it is best to make your own.

Home-made soya bean milk

Cover a pound of soya beans with purified water and leave them soaking all night. In the morning wash them thoroughly by transferring them into a sieve and holding them under running water. Cover with fresh purified water and bring to the boil. If you want to remove the strong soya bean taste which comes through after the milk is made, change the water a couple more times. Drain and grind finely in a food mill. Scrape the pulp with a strong piece of cheesecloth and tie the top together securely. Put into a large saucepan and add four pints of purified warm water. Knead the bag thoroughly so you can see the milk being squeezed out. Pour off the liquid. Repeat the process with the same amount of fresh water and add the original four pints of milk to it. Remove the bag and boil the liquid well, stirring constantly to stop the bottom catching and burning. Cool and store exactly as you would do milk.

Menstruation

The advertising industry, loaded as it is with other sexual references, would con us into believing that bleeding should be sanitised, whitened, neat and discreet. The delicate tampax ballerina in her little white tutu and slippers is a powerful archetype.

I thoroughly disapprove of internal sanitary 'protection' (I use the word advisedly) on several levels. In my experience it heightens a woman's susceptibility to thrush and other vaginal problems; it's not unusual for the last one to be left behind – silly though that may sound. There have also been instances of toxic shock as the result of inserting tampons over abraded skin. Some women have told me they feel tampons soak up all their fluids, not just blood, leaving them feeling dried out completely after menstruation.

Having expressed my preferences, I should also caution women to wipe their bottoms from front to back at all times. If you don't get into this habit and wear a sanitary towel during a period, because it tends to move a little as the body moves, you're in danger of inadvertently spreading unwanted bacteria from the anus to the vagina. Wiping from front to back reduces this risk at all times but especially when bacteria are more easily moved forward by a sanitary towel.

Painful menstruation

Menstruation should not be painful. If cramping is severe at any point, it's because the uterus is heavily burdened with a highly toxic discharge. If blood is bright red it is indicative of poor assimilation of carbohydrates and sugars, if it is dark red and stringy and smelly, it shows the body is overburdened with putrefying protein – meat, eggs and dairy products. Ideally menstruation blood should be a reddish brown.

Pain *immediately before* menstruation may suggest the position of the womb is abnormal – this is more often seen in very thin women who have lost the tone of internal fat and ligament upon which the uterus is suspended. Slant board exercises (see page 288) will help this, as will the exercises mentioned on page 285. If pain precedes menstruation but does not come just before, this may suggest the ovaries are unhealthy, in which case diet should be modified and hot sitz baths taken on alternate nights the week before menstruation is due. All processed and refined foods should be eliminated, and there should be a heavy emphasis on raw and sprouted seeds and nuts, raw organically grown fruits and vegetables, plenty of raw juices daily and supplements of kelp, lecithin and cold-pressed vegetable oils used uncooked as salad dressings. The formula on page 270 will also help, as will raspberry and figwort poultices placed over the abdomen. If pain is felt during the menstrual flow, it means your womb is inflamed and crying out for help, so please seek the help of a medical herbalist immediately.

I've met too many women who've told me about cysts 'the size of a rugby ball', as one patient so graphically put it, who have suffered in silence for years rather than get help. Partly, I suspect, because they've been brought up in the old-fashioned school of thought that a little pain with menstruation is natural and is all part of a women's lot. What nonsense! All menstruation throughout life should be comfortable and easy. If it is not, there is almost certainly something amiss.

For painful, cramping menstruation which occurs at any point during a period
Equal parts of:

> mugwort (*Artemisia vulgaris*)
> cramp bark (*Viburnum opulus*)
> camomile (*Matricaria chamomilla*)
> angelica (*Angelica archargelica*;
> sarsaparilla (*Smilax officinalis*)
> scullcap (*Scutellaria spp*)

Take one cup of this infusion three times a day half an hour before meals with a pinch of cinnamon added to each cup. Do this on a regular daily basis throughout the month. Don't wait for the cramping to start. Also practise the eagle position in yoga and the spinal rock as taught in hatha yoga. If you can't get to a yoga teacher for instructions, the following exercises are worthwhile:

Exercises to relieve menstrual pain
Don't curl up in bed hugging a hot water bottle and feeling sorry for yourself. Force yourself to do the following exercises even though that may be the last thing in the world you feel like.
1.   Lie on your back with your bottom as near to a wall as possible. Prop your feet up against the wall so the soles are flat and the knees a little bent. Stay there for five minutes.
2.   Now move away from the wall and bring one leg up as close to your chin as you can get it. Leave the other on the floor. Grasp the leg you've lifted up with your arms to take the strain and hold that position for two minutes. Then do it using the other leg.
3.   Roll over and get up so that you're resting on your knees and elbows, stretching your head and arms out so that your elbows are on the ground in front of you with your

head between your arms. This is also helpful for those who have pain immediately after intercourse just before a period.

4. Walking, running, swimming or horse riding with regularity also helps. Slothful women get more problems then active ones.

Dysmenorrhoea

For difficult or irregular periods sip cups of mugwort and peppermint tea throughout the day, both with and between meals during the course of your period. Take at least three cups in all. Use a vaginal douche of equal parts of spearmint, sage, elderflowers and marigold, retaining it as long as possible once daily during your period. Use foot or handbaths of the same herbs for the rest of the month.

For excessively heavy menstruation

2 parts shepherd's purse (*Capsella bursa-pastoris*)
1 part lovage (*Levisticum officinale*)
1 part geranium root (*Geranium maculatum*)
1 part squaw vine (*Mitchella repens*)
½ part ginger (*Zingiber officinale*)

Mix as a tincture and take one teaspoon three times daily with meals. Concentrate on iron-rich foods (see page 99) and drink plenty of beetroot juice.

To help the flow during menstruation
Equal parts of:

yellow dock (*Rumex crispus*)
burdock (*Arctium lappa*)
red clover (*Trifolium pratense*)
nettles (*Urtica urens*)
parsley (*Petroselinum spp*)
cinnamon (*Cinnamomun zeylanicum*)

Drink half a cup of the infusion every two hours for the duration of your period.

Metorrhagia

For spotting between periods, take hand or foot baths of equal parts of:

> marshmallow (*Althaea officinalis*)
> blackberry leaves (*Rubus caesius*)
> sage (*Salvia officinalis*)
> hawthorn (*Crataegus oxycantha*)
> garlic (*Allium sativum*)

Ensure there is plenty of calcium in the diet (see page 96). If the condition persists in spite of a good diet and exercise programme and the faithful ingestion of this formula for more than a couple of months, seek the help of a medical herbalist.

Amenorrhoea

No menstruation at all. Take a mustard and ginger warm sitz bath (100°F) on alternate nights. Ensure there's plenty of calcium and iron in the diet (see pages 96 and 99). Adjust the diet to include plenty of hormone-rich foods like banana, wholegrains, sprouted seeds, bee pollen, royal jelly and natural liquorice. Take the following formulation daily on a regular basis for six months:

> 2 parts tansy (*Tanacetum vulgare*)
> 2 parts catnip (*Nepeta cataria*)
> 1 part pennyroyal (*Mentha pulegium*)
> 1 part rosemary (*Rosmarinus officinalis*)
> 1 part liquorice (*Glycyrrhiza glabra*)
> ½ part cinnamon (*Cinnamomum zeylanicum*)

Take two size '00' capsules with each meal. Take each dose with a cup of raspberry tea.

Endometriosis

The endometrium is the blanket that lines the uterus in which the fertilised egg is planted. Poor hygiene before, during or after intercourse (a dirtyish finger inserted into the vagina for example or one that's been inserted in the anus), childbirth, abortion, menstruation, uterine curettage, or carelessly inserted forceps are all means of implanting unfriendly bacteria in the endometrium. Sloppy diet and lifestyle, a wrongly positioned womb, retained placenta, lead poisoning and blood disorders also leave the uterus wide open to infection.

Endometriosis afflicts somewhere between five and ten per cent of women, mainly between the ages of twenty-five and forty-five.

With endometriosis, small fragments of the womb lining may grow in appropriate areas like the ovaries or abdominal cavity.

Symptoms tend to start with the onset of increasingly painful periods after perhaps years of relative comfort. Cyclic bleeding from endometrial tissue (in contrast to menstrual cramps) causes a steady, severe lower abdominal pain which eventually becomes almost constant except in the week following menstruation.

The herbal approach is two-pronged: clear up the infection as speedily as possible and take herbs naturally rich in hormones. Echinacea and goldenseal are excellent antiseptic herbs. Squaw vine, blessed thistle and liquorice are all rich in hormones. So use the following treatments in conjunction with one another.

Douche with equal parts of goldenseal, echinacea, and squaw vine, retaining the douche for as long as possible and for at least twenty minutes. Do this daily. Take the following formulation:

> 3 parts echinacea (*Echinacea angustifolia*)
> 1 part goldenseal (*Hydrastis canadensis*)
> 1 part squaw vine (*Mitchella repens*)
> 1 part blessed thistle (*Carbenia benedicta*)
> 1 part parsley (*Petroselinum spp*)
> 1 part marshmallow (*Althaea officinalis*)
> 1 part cayenne (*Capsicum annum*)
> 1 part liquorice (*Glycyrrhiza glabra*)

Take two size '0' capsules with each meal. If the condition doesn't ease considerably in three months seek the advice of a medical herbalist.

Odd though it may sound, the absence of ovulation and menstruation will effect a cure in a very large number of cases, so for young women who want a family the solution may well be to get pregnant. If there is any recurrence, spacing planned children closer together rather than waiting will also help to prevent flare-ups. In other words, endometriosis may be alleviated by interrupting periodically normal ovarian function and for this reason may also spontaneously improve at the onset of the menopause. Above all, it is a disease which offers the best hope of complete recovery if caught early, so don't hesitate if in doubt. Seek the help of a gynaecologist for confirmation.

Premenstrual tension

If water retention is part of the problem go for the potassium-rich food (see page 102), and of course it goes without saying – no salt. You'll know if you're suffering from water retention because your abdomen will swell up and your ankles and fingers may also become puffy. Your daily vitamins should include 1,000 IUs of vitamin E, provided you do not suffer from hypertension or rheumatic heart complaints, as well as 300 mg B_6 increasing to 500 mg the week before a period, one B complex and two evening primrose oil capsules.

Take the following formulation:

3 parts dandelion (*Taraxacum officinale*)
1 part motherwort (*Leonurus cardiaca*)
1 part wild yam (*Dioscorea villosa*)
1 part lady's slipper (*Cypripedium pubescens*)
1 part borage (*Borago officinalis*)
2 parts horsetail (*Equisetum arvense*)
1 part scullcap (*Scutellaria spp*)
1 part cinnamon (*Cinnamomum zeylanicum*)

Take one size '00' capsule hourly with sips of sarsaparilla tea until the PMT has eased, then reduce to two capsules with each meal. If you keep this treatment up for a minimum of six months on a daily basis, it should alleviate the PMT altogether, at which point you can stop it.

Birth control

There are, as far as I know, no reliable methods of herbal birth control in the West. In China I talked to one of the teams responsible for developing cotton seed oil as a male contraceptive, but it induces liver cancer and until this problem is overcome will obviously not be marketable. The American Red Indians are purported to use some reliable methods of birth control which involve plants, but as at least one of them includes lying half-buried in a trench (not permanently!), they do not seem to be practical for our particular lifestyles.

I'd recommend a mechanical form of birth control like the cap, the sheath or a plastic IUD, not a copper one which tends to leak copper into the system thereby lowering zinc levels. I would not, however, suggest an IUD for women with pelvic or menstrual trouble. I would not recommend the pill in view of its recently acknowledged long-term side-effects.

Coming off the pill

Some say it takes two years to bring the body back to harmony again after a prolonged period of taking the pill. Purify the blood (see page 145), take care of the liver by drinking dandelion coffee and take the following decoction. Equal parts of:

sarsaparilla (*Smilax officinalis*)
blessed thistle (*Carbenia benedicta*)
liquorice (*Glycyrrhiza glabra*)
squaw vine (*Mitchella repens*)
lady's mantle (*Alchemilla vulgaris*)

Take one cup daily for the first six days, resting on the seventh. Then half a cup daily for the next six days. For the third week take one tablespoon daily in sips, then taper the dose off.

Abortion

While there are herbs like tansy and pennyroyal which can be used to induce abortion, I should point out that a herbal abortion is even more traumatic for the body than a medical one and is inadvisable. If you've already had an abortion, the copious use of such herbs as blessed thistle, raspberry, blue vervain and nettles will help restore the glandular system and normalise the womb.

Vaginal infections

These can sometimes be the result of a prolapsed colon, poor pelvic muscle tone and sloppy diet. Look to these and alkalinise the body with lots of potassium broth (see page 102) and a mucusless diet with lots of B complex vitamins.

Thrush

If the itching is unbearable, make a paste of slippery elm and goldenseal using a touch of cider vinegar with the purified water to mix. Spread over the vulva and labia and hold in position with a sanitary towel. Douche once daily with motherwort and goldenseal tea plus one tablespoon cider vinegar, retaining the douche as long as possible.

Alternatively, try applying a poultice of goat's milk yoghurt, holding it in place with a sanitary towel. A word of caution: I've found some women, including myself, react very badly to yoghurt used in this way, so be cautious. Drink lots of oatstraw tea throughout the treatment, at least four cups daily, or take the following formulation. Equal parts of:

> echinacea (*Echinacea angustifolia*)
> goldenseal (*Hydrastis canadensis*)
> periwinkle (*Vinca major*)
> squaw vine (*Mitchella repens*)
> garlic (*Allium sativum*)

Take one size '00' capsule hourly until the yeast infection is under control, then reduce to two with each meal. Ensure the course of herbs lasts for at least twenty-eight days. Your partner must also be treated with equal parts of echinacea, goldenseal, garlic and marshmallow: two size '00' capsules with each meal for the duration of your course of treatment to ensure that the infection is not passed back and forth. Avoid antibiotics which can result in a vaginal fungus infection in susceptible women, and consider coming off the pill and using an alternative contraceptive, because it can cause a sweeter vaginal environment encouraging fungal growth.

Leucorrhoea

Popularly known as 'the whites' because it is a white vaginal discharge which, when it gets out of hand, causes itchiness and pain. Fast for three days on vegetable juices and take half a cup of the following tea hourly:

> 2 parts blue flag (*Iris versicolor*)

2 parts sage (*Salvia officinalis*)
1 part parsley (*Petroselinum spp*)
1 part echinacea (*Echinacea angustifolia*)
1 part dandelion (*Taraxacum officinale*)
1 part goldenseal (*Hydrastis canadensis*)
½ part cinnamon (*Cinnamomum zeylanicum*)

Douche twice daily with equal parts of goldenseal, sage and comfrey made up as an infusion and strained with one tablespoon of cider vinegar added, retaining the douche as long as possible. Once the pain has died down, reduce the douching to once every alternate day and follow the fast outlined on page 160 for a minimum of three days.

Douching

This should only ever be done as part of the treatment for specific gynaecological problems, never for purely aesthetic reasons. The vagina, in health, is self-cleansing and the vulva can be kept clean and sweet with running water and, if necessary, a very mild soap. It is perfectly normal to emit a characteristic but inoffensive odour from the apocrine glands in this area, and each woman has a distinct olfactory signature – the result of differences in glandular activity of the skin, of hormone levels and emotional tension.

When shouldn't you douche?

Douching does *not* stop you getting pregnant. Pregnant women should never douche, nor should they douche for six weeks after delivery. A healthy vagina should not be douched.

How to administer a vaginal douche

Use a gravity-feed douche bag, not a bulb syringe, and fill it with 1¾ litres (2 pt) of well-strained herbal tea which has been allowed to cool to tepid. Hang the bag from a hook on the wall next to the bath, placing it at door handle height. For added comfort heat the bath tub by rinsing it round with hot water first, and lie down. Insert the nozzle about 3.5 cm (1½ in) into the vagina. Release the clamp slowly so that the herbal infusion does not rush into the vagina. Now, using both hands, close the vaginal opening against the nozzle so that the vagina literally becomes flooded with the infusion. You should feel a slight pressure sensation as the vaginal walls expand to accommodate the infusion. When you feel this, turn off the clamp, release your hold and allow the vagina to drain. If you've done it right the infusion will come out in a swoosh. Repeat until the bag is empty.

If you are instructed to retain the douche, grip the muscles you'd normally clench if you were trying to stop yourself urinating when you take the last quarter cup of infusion. Carefully climb out of the bath and adopt one of the inverted yoga positions like the shoulder stand or the pose of tranquillity. Doing this while still in the bath is either, depending on the width of your tub, impossible or dangerous. Hold the pose for as long as you comfortably can and if possible for at least ten minutes. Come out of it slowly and gently. Sit on the toilet or climb back into the bath and let it go. If this proves utterly impossible because your pubococcygeus muscle is too weak, administer the last quarter cup of the douche lying on a slant board and retain for ten minutes.

Gentleness is important at all times. A stream of water which is too forceful can actually flush bacteria from the vagina against the cervix, which could then work their way into the uterine cavity and cause an intra-uterine infection. Always keep your douche bag and syringe scrupulously clean and store it in a sealed bag when not in use.

Cystitis

Fast for three days on vegetable juices and warm vegetable broths. Take as much as you can manage of the following tea – and not less than four cups daily:

> 4 parts marshmallow (*Althaea officinalis*)
> 1 part dandelion (*Taraxacum officinale*)
> 1 part clivers (*Galium aparine*)
> 1 part horsetail (*Equisetum arvense*)
> 1 part borage (*Borago officinalis*)
> ½ part lobelia (*Lobelia inflata*)
> ½ part ginger (*Zingiber officinale*)

Apply hot fomentations of wild thyme with a pinch of ginger to the abdomen.

Contact dermatitis of the vulva

I seem to be seeing more of this in my practice, so I assume it is on the increase. Initially there may only be a slight reddening of the vulva with itching, but if not treated this can lead to labial swelling and the onset of clear blisters which eventually burst and crust over.

First check anything that comes in contact with the vulva – coloured toilet paper, soap, bath additives, soap powder, condoms, vaginal contraceptive foams, tights, feminine sprays, the ingredients in a vaginal douche. Allergic reactions to aspirin, sulphur drugs, phenacetin and some laxatives may also cause vulvar inflammation.

Eliminate the offending agent/s. Soak in basin of cool water with two tablespoons of arrowroot stirred into it. Pat dry gently (no rubbing) and apply a compress of slippery elm, protecting the knickers with a sanitary towel. Once the condition begins to clear, try and let as much air get to the vulva as possible. In the meantime no tights, tight fitting or nylon underwear. Go for loose cotton pants instead.

Genital herpes

The cold sores we get on the mouth are classified as the herpes simplex virus type I, but a closely related virus, herpes simplex virus type II, can affect the vulva, cervix and upper vagina. Because it may be a precursor to cancer of the cervix, it has recently been under close investigation.

Most genital herpes are caused by contact with the type II virus and are picked up during sexual intercourse. But it is possible to transmit the type I virus from a cold sore round the mouth to the genitals during oral sex. Type I virus is not implicated in the development of cervical cancer, but the physical symptoms can be just as distressing and may begin with fever, swollen, tender lymph nodes, excruciating itching and painful blisters along the vulva, and graduate to inflammation around the urethral area, making urination fortuitous. In infections with herpes virus type II, the cervix is apt to be red, irritated and ulcerated, resulting in discharge and vaginal spotting. If you've had no previous encounter with any of the other herpes viruses, like shingles or cold sores, and so have no appropriate antibodies, getting herpes virus type II can be horrendous. The only good news is that most of these symptoms usually fade within two to three weeks.

If pain during urination is excruciating, spraying cold water onto the vulvar area from a shower while doing so will help. Otherwise sit in a bowl of cold water while urinating. Apply cold goat's milk yoghurt compresses for ten minutes at a time six times daily over the affected area. Rinse with a cold shower afterwards and pat on the following tincture. Equal parts of:

goldenseal (*Hydrastis canadensis*)
scullcap (*Scutellaria spp*;
garlic (*Allium sativum*)
lobelia (*Lobelia inflata*)

Patients complain it stings but say that it is preferable to the constant painful itching. Also take sixty drops of the tincture in a little water three times daily with meals. Follow a mucusless diet, that is, one without any refined or processed products, dairy products (except butter and cottage cheese), animal products, salt, sugar, tea, coffee or chocolate.

All women who contact herpes virus type II should have a cervical smear more frequently, and at least once yearly.

Venereal diseases

These have been steadily increasing in this country since the 1960s. In the United States gonorrhoea ranks as the most prevalent communicable disease next to the common cold. So it's no longer safe to assume that venereal disease is only a liability for the sexually promiscuous. On the other hand, just to get the problem into perspective, of every four women who go to a VD clinic in this country, only one of them actually needs treatment for VD. The remainder will be treated for thrush or trichomoniasis or may not need any treatment at all.

Gonorrhoea

This is usually transmitted by sexual intercourse or by intimate contact with the genitalia of an infected person. Very, very occasionally it is possible to pick it up from freshly contaminated towels or sheets. Gonorrhoea does **not** produce symptoms in eighty per cent of all women who are asymptomatic carriers, meaning that although they may themselves never experience the pelvic problems associated with gonorrhoea, they will unknowingly be a source of gonorrhoeal infection to all their sexual contacts. Of the twenty-five per cent who do develop symptoms, an early gonorrhoeal infection begins locally with inflammation of the urethra (which may be so mild many women simply dismiss it as a passing bladder infection). It will spread and involve the cervical glands and produce a purulent yellow discharge. As it is impossible to differentiate this from any other cervical infection, proper lab tests are essential in order to determine the exact nature of the infection.

For this reason I would never treat gonorrhoea herbally. Early and uncomplicated gonorrhoea can readily be treated by antibiotics, bed rest and a strict two month abstinence from sexual intercourse, but if left, the ravages of extensive gonorrhoea can leave a woman a pelvic cripple. So, if in any doubt at all, go to your nearest VD clinic and have the appropriate tests. Don't assume that your doctor will detect or even check for gonorrhoea unless you advise her/him of your concern.

Sex and sexual desire

Anaphrodisiacs

A lot of people treat the subject of substances that dampen sexual desire as a joke, just as they get all leery when I mention the word aphrodisiac. There are lots of reasons why one may want to dampen one's sexual fires – going through a prolonged healing crisis where the body needs plenty of rest, practising natural birth control where a couple may only want to make love during the infertile phases, choosing to live alone and remain celibate.

Avoid garlic, spices, meat, eggs, onion, salt, peppermint, stimulating books or television programmes, and take the following herbal formulation:

2 parts white willow bark (*Salix alba*)
1 part white water lily (*Nymphoeaodorata*)
1 part hops (*Humulus lupulus*)
1 part comfrey root (*Symphytum officinale*)

Make a decoction and take a half cup before each meal.

Failure to reach orgasm

The single most common cause for a woman failing to reach orgasm is inadequate stimulation, but there are other possibilities – underdevelopment of the endocrine and nervous system, diabetes, fear or ignorance, immaturity of the female or male genitalia. Emotional causes require counselling and cooperation from both of you.

Physical causes need individual attention. The following formulation may help. Equal parts of:

> sarsaparilla (*Smilax ornata*)
> saw palmetto (*Serenoa serrulata*)
> damiana (*Turnera diffusa*)
> liquorice (*Glycyrrhiza glabra*)
> cinnamon (*Cinnamomum zeylanicum*)
> prickly ash bark (*Zanthoxylum americanum*)

Mix powdered herbs and take two size '00' capsules with each meal daily for six months only. Omit the liquorice if you have high blood pressure and substitute the same amount of ginger.

Damiana has a marked effect on the sexual system, while prickly ash bark will stimulate the blood circulation. Cinnamon is warming, sarsaparilla is an excellent blood purifier, saw palmetto is rich in natural hormones and liquorice will bolster the adrenal glands and help to counteract stress.

The menopause

Think of this as a time of transition, a new beginning in the middle of adult life, not as a depressing prologue to old age. It's an ideal time to pause and evaluate achievements but, even more important, to plan for the many rewarding years that lie ahead. My lovely adopted aunt went back to school to enjoy the further education she'd been denied as a child and is now a very expert and fulfilled remedial teacher. She could have sat at home and felt sorry for herself as her children took wing and her husband became increasingly immersed in his career, and lost all sense of her own beauty and self-worth. Instead she pushed against the system that conditioned her to see herself in terms of marriage, children and a home and carved out new ground for herself.

Happily only about fifteen per cent of women suffer from true menopausal symptoms – hot flushes, sweats, insomnia, tingling of the extremeties, headaches, occasional palpitations, depressions and fatigue. Hot flushes, though not at all serious, can be disconcerting and at their worst may appear up to fifteen times a day and persist for months. Herbs and foods rich in oestrogen will certainly help.

As the usual course of hormone production during menopause is shifted to the adrenal glands from the ovaries, you may need to take the adrenal formula (see page 256). Premarin, fondly billed as the 'natural' form of oestrogen (presumably because it is collected from the urine of mares) is just as capable of causing dangerous blood clots as the synthetic oestrogens. Vitamin E, up to 1,200 IUs daily, will stimulate the production of oestrogen.

Have your blood pressure checked first, alongside your medical history. It is important to determine whether you ever had rheumatic fever, in which case vitamin E may be contra-indicated, and if you have high blood pressure, it will have to be taken in small doses which are gradually accelerated under supervision.

Make sure you are on the best possible diet with plenty of sprouted seeds, whole grains and bananas, all of which contain oestrogen. Take lots of exercise and acknowledge the fact that you may need a little more relaxation and rest than usual. Take the following oestrogen-rich formulation. Equal parts of:

> blessed thistle (*Carbenia benedicta*)
> squaw vine (*Mitchella repens*)
> lobelia (*Lobelia inflata*)
> raspberry (*Rubus idaeus*)
> cayenne (*Capsicum annum*)
> parsley (*Petroselinum spp*)
> ginger (*Zingiber officinale*)
> marshmallow (*Althaea officinalis*)

Take two size '00' capsules with a cup of sarsaparilla tea with each meal.

Take this as long as you have any uncomfortable menopausal symptoms. If hot flushes become unbearable, take the following formulation as well on the days they occur:

2 parts rosemary (*Rosmarinus officinalis*)
1 part spearmint (*Mentha viridis*)
1 part mugwort (*Artemisia vulgaris*)
1 part St John's wort (*Hypericum perforatum*)
1 part vervain (*Verbena officinalis*)
1 part false unicorn (*Chamaelirium luteum*)

Take one size '00' capsule every two hours with sips of sage tea. Also take hand baths of equal parts of mistletoe leaves, sage, hawthorn and vine leaves.

Mood changes

Women often get tense and irritable during the menopause. This is not surprising if you're seized by devastating hot flushes half the night and have very little uninterrupted sleep, or if you suffer from migraines. Others simply get depressed for no particular reason, and if this is the case the chapter on stress will help. But consider, too, your attitudes towards yourself. If, for example, you're convinced that ageing or perhaps the removal of some female organ makes you less sexually desirable, then your capacity to enjoy lovemaking may naturally be adversely affected. Libido in women is only slightly dependent on the presence of oestrogen and functioning ovaries. Psychological factors are predominant. Women can and should be able to enjoy lovemaking and remain orgasmic as long as they live.

There may be changes in the female genitals – the vulva, vagina and uterus – which make intercourse difficult. Thinning and loss of elasticity in these organs occurs only after a long and significant loss of oestrogen, and in those women it does affect it may not show up for some five to fifteen years. Much depends on how well the ovaries continue to function and how much oestrogen there is in the diet.

The inner walls of the vagina are lined with flattened mucous epithelial cells, some thirty deep, that continually shed, rather like skin cells. In the case of the vagina, harmless resident bacteria help decompose the cellular detritis and while doing so manufacture lactic acid which guards the vagina against harmful bacteria. So the vagina is generally able to look after itself without much conscious help.

Senile vaginas can be helped by vitamin E taken internally and used externally in vaginal bolus form (you'll have to make these yourself), and of course by KY jelly or saliva. The good news is that frequent intercourse keeps the vagina youthful. Lubrication has much less to do with the intensity of stimulation than with its duration, so if you're getting into difficulties, pass that valuable piece of information on to whoever it concerns. However, checking must be done gently. In the post-menopausal woman whose clitoris is relatively more exposed because of labial atrophy, this exquisitely sensitive area will become more vulnerable to direct stimulation during coitus. So stimulation which is too intense is not at all exciting, indeed it can be distressing and painful.

Prolapse of the uterus
Take three cups of the following tea daily for a minimum of nine months. One part of each of:

> lady's mantle (*Alchemilla vulgaris*)
> nettles (*Urtica urens*)
> St John's wort (*Hypericum perforatum*)

Also practise strengthening the P-C muscles. To do this, pretend you want to urinate urgently but need to hold back the flow. Lift and clench the internal muscles that will enable you to do this. Now let them go. Now clench, hold firmly and let go at a rhythmic and comfortable pace. Do this 200 times daily. You won't be able to do them all at once, it'll be too exhausting. But once the P-C muscle gets stronger you'll manage forty or fifty at a time.

Also do your slant board exercises daily.

CHAPTER 11

Ageing

Many of the changes I see in elderly people are psychological not physiological. You only begin to atrophy once you've lost your enthusiasm for life, once you've stopped planning for the future, once you feel you've got nothing worthwhile to contribute. But there's not much point in putting all your zest and love into life if your body can't keep up with you. So simply refuse to atrophy. Get fit, then stay fit. Ageing, like pregnancy, isn't a disease, so don't expect illness or give into it if it comes.

Exercise

The greatest deficiency among the elderly is not diet but exercise. Make it something you like – dancing, swimming, rambling, golf – and indulge regularly. One of my patients celebrated her sixty-seventh year by swimming sixty-seven lengths in the local baths, and she intended to *increase* this by one length yearly, not decrease it as the years advanced. Regular exercise will help you counteract weakness, stiffness and loss of balance, and so radically cut down the chance of having a fall or an accident due to lack of confidence. If the exercise is a group activity, so much the better, as it will expand your horizons, though that doesn't mean to say you can't go for nature rambles by yourself (as one of my favourite patients does – indeed he'll be showing me how to bleed birch trees this spring, which I'm looking forward to).

One of the major causes of senile dementia is a declining circulation to the brain, and sustained exercise keeps the blood circulating properly. Slant board exercises are particularly beneficial for getting blood of oxygen to the brain. There are a few instances in which slant boards are not advisable – for example, hypertension, stomach ulcers, tendency to haemorrhage, some tubercular conditions, appendicitis, or cancer in the pelvic cavity – so check with your medical herbalist or doctor first.

Slant board exercises

Choose a good strong piece of wood about the width of a door so that it can easily accommodate your shoulders when you lie on it; it should be at least six inches longer than your height. Ensure there are no splinters on the board and that you can raise it firmly at one end with no risk of it falling or sliding off. I have a wooden ledge on the underside of mine which hooks firmly over the empty bottom shelves of a sturdy book case. Begin with a three inch slope and gradually, at your own pace, increase this to twenty-four inches or about chair seat height. Do these exercises for five minutes at mid-afternoon, and for five minutes just before bed, not counting an initial five minutes spent simply lying on the flat board, head at the lower end, letting gravity reposition your insides, with your arms by your sides. This will gradually correct any prolapses of internal organs like the transverse colon, stomach or uterus, or will protect against such collapse.

1. With your head at the lower end, breathe in slowly, raise your arms and stretch them above your head, reaching right back so that you touch the floor behind you. When you get there, breathe out and hold for a few seconds. Breathe in and bring your arms back. Rest and then repeat ten times.

2. Now, with your arms by your sides, breathe out fully and suck your stomach muscles in. Hold for a few seconds, then snap them out, at which point you'll automatically breathe in again. Relax. Repeat ten times.

3. Give yourself a stomach massage (see page 145), or if this is initially too strenuous, try rolling a small ball (about the size of a tennis ball) over your lower colon, pressing deeply as you follow its path from right to left in a big clockwise circle.

4. Holding on to the sides of the board firmly, slowly bend your knees so they're resting on your chest. Don't worry if you can't do this fully at first. It'll come in time. Now turn your head fully from side to side, five times on each side. Then, if you can, lift your head slightly and rotate it, first

clockwise, then anti-clockwise, three times each, then slowly replace your legs.

5. Lift your legs vertically. It doesn't matter if you bend at the knees slightly. Rotate outwards in circles ten times, first with one foot, then with the other, then both together.

6. Rest now, because that's quite strenuous. When you've got your breath back, lift your legs up again, this time keeping them as straight as you can at the knees. Bring them up to a vertical position both together. Now lower them slowly back to the board. Repeat four times.

7. Now cycle with your legs in the air working up to twenty-five times eventually.

8. Now relax, and as you get your breath back, squeeze all the muscles in your face hard, then let them go, and feel the tension flooding from your face. As your breathing slows down to normal, feel the tension seeping out of your body. Relax and rest for five minutes minimum, letting the recharged blood circulate into your head. Get up slowly.

These exercises are particularly good for those with eye problems, falling hair or any untoward hair condition, sinus problems, ear problems or indeed any inflammation above the shoulders, varicosity, prolapse of the abdominal organs, and they will help failing memory, dizziness (provided it's not the result of high blood pressure), and fatigue.

To further help your brain do some deep breathing exercises (see page 153), preferably out of doors. If it's cold, wrap up well. If you're disabled, move your wheelchair next to an open window. One of the reasons memory fails is insufficient oxygen to the brain: the other is insufficient use. So exercise your brain with as much enthusiasm as you exercise your body.

Formulation to help the brain

Equal parts of the following finely powdered herbs:

rosemary (*Rosmarinus officinalis*)
cayenne (*Capsicum annum*)
Siberian ginseng (*Panax ginseng*)
gota kola (*Centella asiatica*)
parsley (*Petroselinum spp*)
alfalfa (*Medicago sativa*)

Take two size '0' capsules with each meal.

Diet

It's a great temptation to eat convenience food if you're living alone or only cooking for two. Or worse still, hardly to eat at all. This is particularly common in people who are grieving. The elderly are known to be chronically short of vitamin C, calcium and vitamins A and D. As you grow older, the amount of food you need to maintain your ideal body weight decreases by five per cent for every ten years past the age of twenty, but please note that there is no correlative reduction of the need for protein, vitamins, minerals and amino acids. In other words, junk foods rob you of proportionally more nutrition as you grow older, even if you don't eat more of them. A sobering thought.

So how do you begin if you haven't been on a natural diet all your life? The answer is very gradually and gently. If you fill your beaten-up digestive tract with whole grains and lots of fresh fruit and vegetables when you've been used for years to eating tinned foods and refined products, you'll have an internal riot on your hands. So if you're switching take one item at a time on a weekly basis. Begin, for example, by cutting out salt. Then the next week move over to whole grains. If you're introducing bran for the first time, try one teaspoon at a time at first. In the third week try a small side salad with your midday meal. Within four or five months you'll have changed onto a wholefood diet and hopefully be experimenting with it and enjoying it. To ensure you're getting all the vitamins and minerals you need, take the following herbs as a supplement.

Vitamin/mineral supplement

Equal parts of the following herbs, finely powdered:

> parsley root and/or leaf (*Petroselinum spp*)
> alfalfa (*Medicago sativa*)
> nettles (*Urtica urens*)
> horsetail (*Equisetum arvense*)
> camomile flowers (*Matricaria chamomilla*)
> watercress (*Nasturtium officinale*)
> garlic (*Allium sativum*)

cayenne (*Capsicum annum*)
dandelion (*Taraxacum officinale*)
rosehips (*Rosaceae*)
Irish moss (*Chondrus crispus*)
kelp (*Fucus spp*)
meadow-sweet (*Spiraea ulmaria*)

Take half a level teaspoon three times daily stirred with a little black strap molasses at the beginning of each meal.

If you simply can't eat because you're ill or grieving, take lots of slippery elm, freshly pressed juices and this vitamin supplement. If whole grains or vegetables are a problem because it hurts to chew them, *don't* make this an excuse for avoiding them. Liquidise the vegetables into soups or press out their juices and have them that way. Mill the grains and nuts by pounding them in a pestle and mortar or grinding them in a coffee mill.

Alcohol in moderation is fine, but don't come to rely on it because you feel depressed or lonely, and always take it with meals or just before a meal. A glass of sherry before a meal or a glass of good wine with one stimulates the gastric juices (hence St Paul's advice 'to use a little wine for thy stomach's sake'). It also reduces the activity of the viral inhabitants of the intestines, so it's a mild bacteriocide, and it helps the circulation by dilating the blood vessels and reducing blood pressure. Recent American studies have shown that moderate drinkers tend to live longer on average than either heavy drinkers or total abstainers. But alcohol *must* be taken in moderation, sipped slowly and linked with food.

Smoking is absolutely out. I don't have to read you the riot act about what it does to you, I'm sure, but just remember you have a much higher chance of dying earlier than you need to from lung cancer, bronchitis, emphysema or heart disease if you do. And a pretty high chance of doing so even if you don't but live with someone who does. Try and protect your lungs by not breathing in car fumes, and if you live in a city get out to the countryside or an open park as much as possible.

Finally think about how you look. How do you present yourself to the world? Beauty and vitality isn't just the prerogative of youth. One of my patients never fails to dazzle me with her lively hairstyle, her charming smile and her well-pressed, colour-coordinated clothes.

If you can't find advice or the remedy you need in the following section, look up your ailment in the index. I've covered the areas I know my own elderly patients find problematical, but it is by no means comprehensive and the more serious complaints are listed in Chapter 10.

Hair loss

A receding hairline is a problem that seems to preoccupy many men, but baldness in women, though unusual, does happen.

If you want to go really mad, the alternative step to camouflage is the radical step of shaving it all off, which looks deliberate and expresses a lot of self-confidence. After all, some men look terrific bald – Yul Brynner and Telly Savalas to name but two. But you have to have a well-shaped cranium to get away with it. This is not a step, I'll readily admit, which would appeal to most women!

Look at your diet and ensure it is particularly rich in the B vitamins as well as A and C, iron, iodine and copper. Iodine is especially important as it is needed for the proper functioning of the thyroid gland, which in turn encourages efficient scalp circulation (see page 98). A good haircut helps to redirect the eye away from the bald area to where the hair really is. There's nothing worse, to my mind, than seeing a man with a long piece of hair plastered across his bald patch.

As with every health problem, prevention is better than cure and liable to save more falling hair. So do your slant board exercises daily. Encourage efficient scalp circulation by massaging it daily with your fingertips and a few drops of essential oil of rosemary in almond oil. Tense your fingers and start at the nape of your neck, working forward to your forehead in small rotating circles. Use a brush with well-spaced natural bristles with rounded ends and a flexible rubber base, and a non-metal wide-toothed comb, and wash them daily. Shampoo your hair with a warm decoction of soapwort (*Saponaria officinalis*) and rinse with a decoction of rosemary or nettles or southernwood with a few drops of cider vinegar. These decoctions can also be dabbed liberally onto the roots of the hair every day using a piece of cotton wool.

Eyes

Exercises for the eyes

Rub your palms together hard so that the friction generates some heat. Cup your palms over your eyes, fingers pointing up to the hairline. Let your eyes bask in the warmth and darkness of the palms. Stay like this until the heat has dissipated. Now trail your fingers gently across your eyes from the inner corners to the temples. Repeat the whole procedure five times.

Pretend you have a very large clock right in front of your eyes with the numbers of the hours painted on the extreme outside of the circle. Starting at twelve o'clock, very slowly move your eyes from one hour to the next, pausing for a second at each number, and following a clockwise direction. Keep your head immobile. When you reach twelve o'clock, stop. Rest. Then go backwards moving your eyes in an anti-clockwise direction. Gently move your head and neck through the largest circle shape you can manage, keeping your shoulders steady. Don't strain and don't exaggerate your movements. At first your neck muscles may be so tense you can only sketch a small circle; but practice will help loosen up the muscles and make the exercise easier. This will improve your vision by increasing the circulation to the optic nerve and help to ease shoulder strain.

Lotion to strengthen the eyes

> 1 tbsp rue flowers (*Ruta graveolens*)
> 1 tsp fennel seeds, bruised (*Foeniculum officinale*)
> 1 tsp eyebright leaves (*Euphrasia officinalis*)
> 1 tsp white wine
> 120 ml (4 fl oz) mineral water

Put all the ingredients in a sterilised glass bowl and place over a pot of boiling water. Cover with a clean china plate. Allow the lotion to heat gently for two hours, remembering to top up the boiling water in the pot from time to time. Allow to cool still covered. Strain through coffee filter paper. Immediately store in a sterilised container. Use this lotion as an eye bath to bathe the eyes twice daily. It'll last two to three days. Then make some more fresh lotion.

When using an eye bath, tilt the head well back. Rock it from side to side then, keeping the head steady, roll the eyes first clockwise and then anti-clockwise. Use fresh lotion for each eye, rinsing the eye bath cup out in between.

Ears

Ringing in the ears

First look to cleansing the blood and the bowel (see Chapter 5). Then improve the circulation, because a lot of that ringing is often due to poor circulation.

Make up the following tincture:

> 1 part garlic (*Allium sativum*)
> 1 part sage (*Salvia officinalis*)
> 1 part hawthorn (*Crataegus oxycantha*)
> 1 part dandelion (*Taraxacum officinale*)
> 2 parts motherwort (*Leonurus cardiaca*)
> 1 part cayenne (*Capsicum annum*)

Make as a standard tincture and take fifteen drops (internally with your food) three times daily. Footbaths and handbaths using the above ingredients are also helpful.

All ear infections or pain must be treated promptly by a professional, otherwise you risk permanent damage, possibly even deafness.

Dr Christopher's oil and tincture combination

This formula is designed to improve poor equilibrium and sharpen hearing. Every night, with an eye dropper, put four drops of garlic oil into each ear. Then add four drops of the following tincture. Equal parts of:

> black cohosh (*Cimicifuga racemosa*)
> blue cohosh (*Caulophyllum thalictroides*)
> blue vervain (*Verbena officinalis*)

scullcap (*Sculleratia spp*)
lobelia (*Lobelia inflata*)

Plug each ear with cotton wool. On the seventh day gently syringe out the ears with half-and-half distilled water and cider vinegar. Please try and get professional medical help to do this. If this is not available be sure to use a little bulb, not a great big ear syringe, otherwise you may puncture your ear drum, and wield it very carefully and gently. Keep up this treatment for a month. Also massage the tincture into the medulla oblongata situated at the base of the skull and into the area behind the ears.

Mouth

If your gums start bleeding with only the slightest pressure, go to your dentist post-haste. Meanwhile ensure you're getting lots of vitamins A, D and C. 25,000 IUs of A, 1,000 IUs of D, and 3-4 g of C. Rinse your mouth out repeatedly with decoctions of bistort, tormentil or white oak bark. Rub the gums with a paste of pounded magnesia powder and gallunt. Do not swallow this because it tastes absolutely terrible. Spit it out.

Loose teeth and spongy gums

Again look to your diet and ensure you have an abundance of Vitamin A, D and C. Clean the teeth with a soft brush and the following tooth powder:

Equal parts of bistort, bayberry, sage and orris. Rinse afterwards with a double strength (ie 2 oz/1 pt) decoction of bistort. Then surround the gums round the loose teeth with powdered white oak bark and try, if you can, to leave it in all night. If you swallow a bit it doesn't matter. Continue the treatment till the gums have firmed up.

If you want to continue to enjoy life to the full, savour every present moment passionately, enjoy your exercise, learn to breathe properly and relax deeply, nourish yourself appropriately and try not to take any drugs if at all possible. Vast numbers of elderly and, indeed, middle-aged people lack vitality because they are permanently drugged. You've read this book and you now know there is a better way to help yourself. Use it.

Appendix

Good-quality dried herbs are available by mail order from:

Neal's Yard Remedies,
5 Golden Cross, Cornmarket Street, Oxford, OX1 3EU. Telephone 01865 245436, Fax (same as telephone).

Baldwins,
173 Walworth Road, London SE17 1RW. (Personal callers welcome Tuesday to Saturday). Telephone 0171 703 5550, Fax 0171 252 6261.

Herbs in quantities of at least 1 kg are available from:

Herbal Apothecary,
103 The High Street, Syston, Leicester, LE7 1BQ. Telephone 0116 2602690, Fax 0116 2602757.

A wide selection of powdered herbs, herbal tinctures, herbal creams and ointments as well as encapsulated herbs are available from:

Kitty Campion,
The Natural Health and Iridology Centre,
25 Curzon Street, Basford, Newcastle under Lyme, Staffordshire, ST5 0PD. Telephone 01782 711592, Fax 01782 713274.

BioCare Ltd,
54 Northfield Road, Kings Norton, Birmingham, B30 1JH. Telephone 0121 433 3727, Fax 0121 433 3879.

Bioforce (UK) Ltd,
Olympic Business Park, Dundonald, Ayrshire, KA2 9BE. Telephone 01563 851177.

Cytoplan Limited,
St Peters Chambers, 40 St Peters Street, Tiverton, Devon, EX16 6NR. Telephone 01884 258080, Fax 01884 255333.

Gerard House Limited,
475 Capability Green, Luton, LU1 3LU. Telephone 01582 482929, Fax 01582 484941.

D. Napier & Sons,
18 Bristo Place, Edinburgh, Scotland, EH1 1EZ. Telephone 0131 255 5542, Fax 0131 220 3981.

Nelson & Co Ltd,
77 Duke Street, London W1. (Creams available to personal callers only.) Telephone 0171 495 2404, 0181 788 7888.

Mail order service is available from:

Nelson & Co Ltd,
5 Endeavour Way, London, SW19 9UH. Telephone 0181 946 8527, Fax 0181 946 6202.

An excellent range of essential oils is available in individual dropper bottles from:

Butterbur & Sage Ltd,
PO Box 41, Southall, Middlesex, UB1 3BZ.

Excellent-quality vitamins and minerals including amino-acids are available from:

Nature's Best,
PO Box 1, Tunbridge Wells, Kent, TN2 3EQ. Telephone 01892 539595, Fax 01892 515863.

Larkhall Green Farm,
225 Putney Bridge Road, London, SW15 2PY. Telephone 0181 874 1130, Fax (same as telephone).

Rescue Remedy and other Bach flower remedies as well as Rescue Remedy Cream are available from:

The Doctor Edward Bach Centre,
Mount Vernon, Sotwell, Wallingford, Oxfordshire, OX10 0PX. Telephone 01491 834 678, Fax 01491 825 022.

Nelson's make a superb marigold cream together with ones for bruises, burns and chilblains. The Company have a shop at:

77 Duke Street, London, where you can call and collect these and other natural remedies. Telephone 0171 495 2404.

Excellent quality Spirulina farmed from clean seas around New Zealand as well as organic aloe vera juice can be obtained directly from:

Xynergy Health Products,
Ash House, Stedham, Midhurst, West Sussex, GU29 0PT. Telephone 01730 813642, Fax 01730 815109.

HERB GROWING

The British Herb Trade Association provides guidance on herb gardening which includes the setting-up of a herb garden, the whereabouts of good quality herbs, advice on tending a herb garden and useful names and addresses for further information. A 'Herb Pack' is available at a reasonable price and occasionally gardening courses are also available. For information write to:

The Chairman,
Hereford Herbs, Remenham House, Ocley Pychard, Herefordshire, HR1 3RB.

Many of the people who belong to the British Herb Trade Association will supply seedlings and seeds by post and these can also be collected in person. These include:

Iden Croft Herbs,
Frittenden Road, Staplehurst, Kent, TW12 0DH. Telephone 01580 891432, Fax 01580 892416.

Oak Cottage Herb Farm,
Nesscliffe, Nr Shewsbury, Shropshire. Telephone 01743 741262

Herb gardens are a pleasure to visit as well as being educational and are as varied and as interesting as their owners. A list of herb gardens throughout Britain is available from:

The Herb Society,
134 Buckingham Palace Road, London. Telephone 0171 823 5583.

Organic vegetables are available from growers who are members of:

The Soil Association,
86/88 Colston Street, Bristol, BS1 5BB. Telephone 0117 9290661, Fax 0117 9252504.
Enema and douche kits and natural skin brushes as well as many of the formulations in this book are available from:

Kitty Campion,
The Natural Health and Iridology Centre, 25 Curzon Street, Basford, Newcastle under Lyme, Staffordshire, ST5 0PD. Telephone 01782 711592, Fax 01782 713274.

Many Chinese supermarkets stock Chinese bamboo steamers. Water filters are generally available from health food stores and some chemists. An excellent range of juicers, ionizers and trampolines are available from:

The Wholistic Research Company (UK),
Bright Haven, Robin's Lane, Lolworth, Cambridge, CB3 8HH. Telephone 01954 781074.

EQUIPMENT

Enema and douche kits and natural skin brushes as well as many of the formulations in this book are available from:

Kitty Campion,
The Natural Health and Iridology Centre, 25 Curzon Street, Basford, Newcastle under Lyme, Staffordshire, ST5 0PD. Telephone 01782 711592, Fax 01782 713274.

Many Chinese supermarkets stock Chinese bamboo steamers. Water filters are generally available from health food stores and some chemists. An excellent range of juicers, ionizers and trampolines are available from:

The Wholistic Research Company (UK),
Bright Haven, Robin's Lane, Lolworth, Cambridge, CB3 8HH. Telephone 01954 781074.

HERBAL COURSES

Kitty Campion is the Director of the College of Herbs & Natural Healing, UK. It is the European branch of the American School founded over half a century ago in Utah, USA, by Dr Christopher, America's foremost wholistic herbalist. It trains students to be herbal practitioners, awarding the advanced American qualification of Master Herbalist. It also offers training in the diagnostic skill of Iridology and in body work including traditional Thai Healing massage and all of these qualifications are designed to equip practitioners to practice on a professional level. The College also holds on-going advanced courses yearly throughout its therapies for all professional practitioners.

The College of Herbs & Natural healing is also a founder member of the Pan European Herbal Alliance, an umbrella organisation for all the established herbal schools in Europe. Kitty Campion will be happy to direct you to any of these schools for professional training. As in every profession, the skill of Medical Herbalists and Iridologists will vary. Choose someone who fits into your life-style. You may go for the leather-thonged, red-shirted naturopath breathing fire and brimstone and carrot or you may prefer the white-coated quieter approach. But whoever you choose, look for and expect professionalism. The best way to make a choice is to talk to other patients working with the practitioner you have in mind. By their results shall you know them. If a patient has been going to see a practitioner for the last two years there is something wrong. This obviously means the disease is not being helped. Choose someone who specialises in one field only. The jack-of-all-trades and master of none with a wall littered with weekend course certificates is no good to you. Be prepared to work with someone who will open-mindedly refer you onto another branch of naturopathy if necessary. Herbalism isn't the panacea of all ills. Neither is acupuncture or osteopathy though some practitioners evidently believe so!

The only patients Kitty Campion tends to see for more than five or six visits are those with deeply entrenched diseases like multiple sclerosis or diabetes. She does, however, also like to see patients for a yearly check-up on a preventative basis.

Kitty Campion conducts residential natural healing weekend workshops in the UK and the USA showing participants how to use herbs to help the body heal itself, as well as basic introductory classes to yoga and to vegan cookery. These classes are designed for anyone wanting to help themselves and their family and friends to maintain good health safely and simply and no qualifications are awarded. Kitty Campion also offers a home study course on the basics of natural healing assisted by audio and visual aids and workbooks.

OTHER USEFUL ADDRESSES

At the time of writing, the Department of Health is threatening the survival of more than 1,000 natural medicines. If you feel strongly that the Department of Health should not be allowed to do this, please join the Natural Medicine Society. Ordinary membership currently costs £5.

Natural Medicine Society,
Market Chambers, 15A Market Place, Heanor, Derbyshire, DE75 7AA. Telephone 01773 710002.

The Institute for Complementary Medicine,
15 Tavern Quay, Plough Way, Surrey Quay, London, SE16 1QZ. Telephone 0171 237 5165, Fax 0171 237 5175. The Institute promotes natural therapies and methods of healing.

For help with post-natal illness contact:

The Association of Post-natal Illness,
25 Jerdan Place, Fulham, London, SW6 1BE. Telephone 0171 386 0868.

BODY ALIGNMENT

Pilates technique, a well-worked-out unique system of body realignment is available on personal application to:

Alan Herdman,
Pilates Technique, 17 Homer Row, London W1H 1HU. Telephone 0171 723 9953, Fax 0171 354 4082.

The Alexander technique which teaches balance, posture and movement appropriate for everyday activities is at:

The Society of Teachers of the Alexander Technique,
20 London House, 226 Fulham Road, London, SW10 9EL. Telephone 0171 351 0828.

Index